Toward Equity in Quality in Mathematics Education

Murad Jurdak

Toward Equity in Quality
in Mathematics Education

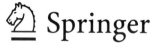 Springer

Murad Jurdak
Department of Education
American University of Beirut (AUB)
Beirut, Lebanon
jurdak@aub.edu.lb

ISBN 978-1-4419-0557-4   e-ISBN 978-1-4419-0558-1
DOI 10.1007/978-1-4419-0558-1
Springer Dordrecht Heidelberg London New York

Library of Congress Control Number: 2009931583

Printed on acid-free paper

Springer is part of Springer Science+Business Media (www.springer.com)

To

My firstborn son Eid whose life was cut short at 10 years by a car bomb during the senseless civil war in Lebanon.

The memory of my parents who struggled hard to give me the start I needed for making it in life.

Preface

The first decade of this century witnessed the emergence of a new goal, namely providing equal opportunity to quality education for all students. This goal is becoming a challenge to the international community, to national governments, schools, educators and parents. Mathematics is considered as a major core school subject and is at the center of this challenge.

Toward Equity in Quality in Mathematics Education is a comprehensive book dedicated to the issues of equity and quality in mathematics education and through it I hope to fill a gap in the literature in this respect. This book is based on and driven by four premises. The first premise is that mathematics education is a purposeful collective human activity enacted in a specific social-cultural context and constitutes a complex multifactor system. The second premise is that inequities in mathematics education result from multiple interactions among the factors of the aforementioned system and are not simply 'achievement gaps' associated with isolated factors such as gender, ethnicity, or socioeconomic status. The third premise is that inequities occur in nested hierarchical systems of mathematics education i.e. among students in the same class, among schools in the same country, and among countries at the global level. Hence, the inequities in one system are likely to impact those in other systems. The fourth premise is that viewing inequities as interactions in a multifactor system render them amenable to change by changing policies or practices while taking into consideration the complexity of the nested hierarchical systems in which they occur. Using the lens of these premises, this book attempts to recast and synthesize existing research on equity and quality in mathematics education (Part I) and to analyze and interpret TIMSS 2003 data (Part II) from that perspective.

Part I, titled *Equity in Quality in Mathematics Education: Perspectives and Contexts* addresses equity in quality from a personal perspective by telling the story of my journey to equity in quality in mathematics education as well as from the historical perspective of the evolution of equity and quality notions in each of education and mathematics education. Using the construct of Engeström's activity system, Part I also examines and synthesizes equity and quality research in school, country and global contexts.

Part II, titled *Equity in Quality in Mathematics Education: Across Countries Comparisons Based on TIMSS 2003 Data*, presents an analysis of TIMSS 2003 contextual data across a sample of 18 countries. This analysis attempts to identify, compare, and interpret student, teacher, school, and country related variables which account for variation in mathematics achievement. Part II concludes with an epilogue containing proposals for moving toward equity in quality.

It would be impossible to acknowledge all those many individuals who have contributed to this book as it is an accumulation of professional experiences spanning my whole career. I am indebted to all my students, colleagues, and friends who have contributed directly or indirectly to this work. My thanks also goes to my daughter Hania, my son Raja, and my sister-in-law Samira Shami for their help in technical matters. My great appreciation goes to my wife, Muna, herself a mathematics educator, who acted as a critical reader through all the stages of preparing the manuscript. She provided valuable comments regarding the content, clarity of meaning, and language use. I would also like to acknowledge the contribution of Ms Nada Rahhal who did the statistical analysis and the preparation of the graphs.

I specially would like to acknowledge my university, the American University of Beirut (AUB) for granting me a one-semester leave to enable me to finish writing this book. Last but not least, I would like to thank the Department of Education at AUB for providing services of graduate students and research assistants to support my work all through.

This book was an opportunity for me to use equity in quality as a context for reflecting on my professional career and making coherent meaning of the many professional experiences I have had. I hope the reader will enjoy this book as much as I enjoyed my journey to get to it.

Beirut, Lebanon   Murad Jurdak

Contents

Part I

Equity in Quality in Mathematics Education:
Contexts and Perspectives

1

My Journey Toward Equity in Quality

This chapter is a personal reconstruction of memories of thoughts and events that occurred through my life and that relate to issues of quality, equity, and mathematics education. They are not based on any existing record, such as logs and diaries, but rather on my retrospective interpretation of the meanings of these thoughts and events from my perspective now, since I was not sure what they meant when they actually occurred, or whether they had any meaning at all then! This reconstruction spans my life starting from childhood, as early as I can remember, and up to the present. Of course I shall be carefully selective and I shall choose the thoughts and events that represent turning points in the development of my thinking on equity and quality.

The story of my journey towards equity in quality will be divided into six sections representing the chronological evolution of my thinking regarding these issues:

1. The Nineteen Fifties: The School Years
2. The Nineteen Sixties: The University Years
3. The Nineteen Seventies: The Start of a Career in Mathematics Education
4. The Nineteen Eighties: The Beginning of the Social Turn
5. The Nineteen Nineties: Problem Solving in School and Outside
6. The Present: Reflecting on the Past and Looking Ahead

1.1 The Nineteen Fifties: The School Years

I come from a town in South Lebanon about 100 km south east of Beirut. The town residents may be described according to the standards in the nineteen fifties, as mainly middle class, including merchants, landowners, and professionals with a minority working class of soldiers, artisans, and workers. My father was an artisan/small contractor, and as such my family was a working class family. My mother, who had a high school diploma from an American

M. Jurdak, *Toward Equity in Quality in Mathematics Education*,
DOI 10.1007/978-1-4419-0558-1_1,
© Springer Science+Business Media, LLC 2009

missionary school and had a working knowledge of English, was considered to be an educated individual according to the standards of the time. My family, especially my mother, had high educational expectations for the children, particularly for me, being the only male child in the family.

My town was known to be the educational hub of the district. Its many schools, which were all tuition-based and affiliated with Christian organizations, attracted many students of diverse socioeconomic and religious backgrounds, from neighboring villages and towns. In the late forties, my school was established by a group of Lebanese notables living in the west, and as such was the first non-sectarian, non-profit school, with no religious affiliation whatsoever. At that time, hardly 10 years after Lebanon became independent from the French mandate, there was no public school in the town.

In the early primary grades, I do not remember being aware of my socioeconomic status. As I became more conscious of my socioeconomic status, I started to develop a sense of empowerment. Now that I can analyze it from my present perspective, I can trace that sense of empowerment to at least two factors. First, from home, I brought to school a resilient motivation to excel, as the only way up the socioeconomic ladder for me and for my family. Second, I did distinguish myself at school through academic achievement in all subjects, including mathematics, and this drive to excel became obsessive to the point that I became determined to achieve the highest average in class in every subject.

Given this head start, I started to realize that the personal capital I owned (my distinguished ability for academic achievement) and my home capital (attitudes and values) were valuable to the point that the principal of the school, a compassionate and visionary educator, allowed me to continue in school even after I informed him that my family would not be able to pay tuition anymore. In fact, my capital counterbalanced any inequities that may have arisen because of my socioeconomic status.

I would like to pause here at my experience from the perspective of the human capital as proposed by Bourdieu et al. (1994). The construct of the home habitus (home culture) has a lot of value, theoretically and empirically, however, it may lead to misinterpretations when it is used to label situations like the 'working class home habitus'. Although the attributes of the 'home habitus of the working class' may be similar across many situations in the same country or even across countries, they also have differences due to the specificity of each situation. The personal stories of many, mine included, may be looked at as atypical instances of the 'working class home habitus'. Throughout my school years, not only had I not felt disadvantaged because of my socioeconomic status, but on the contrary, I felt proud of being a disadvantaged student.

During my school years, my conception of mathematics passed through several phases. In primary grades we studied mathematics in Arabic and used locally-authored textbooks. On the one hand, mathematics seemed to me, at the time to be a collection of useful techniques in which speed and correctness were critical. On the other hand, math included solving challenging word problems, which were not intended for use in the real world as much as they were a context for exercising our mental abilities and using the mathematical techniques we learned. In the primary grades, the focus was arithmetic and geometry, the study of the latter limited to identifying shapes and finding the areas and volumes through formulas.

As we moved to middle school, my conception of mathematics started to expand because of the introduction of both algebra and the rudimentary axiomatic method and proof in geometry. Algebra was a new turn for me for many reasons. First, we shifted from learning mathematics in Arabic to English and suddenly the English alphabet letters assumed new meaning of their own. They were not only sounds but also unknowns (variables were not in fashion then!). Second, we started to use heavy, hard-cover and neatly printed British mathematics textbooks, and that was a symbol of our promotion to a higher status. The rudimentary axiomatic method of Euclidean geometry was also a breakthrough for me as I looked at it aesthetically, at that time, as a beautiful systematic process of building a logical foundation for something I already intuitively knew. The introduction of proof was intriguing for me, because it gave one a sense of security, that could not be challenged. However, at the beginning, my understanding of proof was formal and limited to theorems.

1.2 The Nineteen Sixties: The University Years

Coming from a low socioeconomic status would have been a barrier to join a private university, let alone the most expensive one. The 'home capital' I carried and my school success story helped me land a full scholarship at the American University of Beirut (AUB), the elitist and prestigious university in the Middle East. The requirement of my scholarship was that the field of study be a developmental one, such as agriculture, education, or public administration. My school grades made me eligible to be accepted in any field of study. However, I chose math as a major, and to satisfy the requirements of my scholarship I had to study for a teaching diploma, along with my Bachelor's degree in math. Though I would have preferred literature, I eventually chose mathematics as my subject because of my belief that it was regarded by society as the most prestigious of all other school subjects both intellectually and economically.

At AUB I had my first true experience with a multi-cultural society. In the nineteen sixties, the AUB student body, which had a representation of over 60 nationalities, was a true multi-cultural community with students coming from many countries such as Iran, Afghanistan, Sudan, Cyprus, most Arab countries, and many European and American countries. The professors also represented a multi-cultural mix. This experience taught me the positive side of living in a multi-cultural community with people of different colors, languages, and cultures.

During my undergraduate study, I experienced some changes in my conception of mathematics. Earlier, I had considered mathematics as a haven where one could enjoy reasoning and problem solving without any accountability to reality. This conception was somehow shaken by my experiences in the science courses, especially physics, which I had to take as a requirement for my program. I started to appreciate the power of mathematics in relation to reality as represented in physics-a power which allows the scientist to use mathematics to model reality, solve problems within the mathematical model, and consequently apply it to solve problems in physics. Though I felt empowered by this idea of modeling in physics, I also was disturbed by the lack of both security and absolute validity that existed in mathematics.

A second experience which impacted my conception of mathematics was the idea of mathematical structure as I experienced it in modern algebra and topology. Although the ideas of modeling and mathematical structure seem too paradoxical to coexist in one's belief system, I learned to think of them as complementary to one another: The more abstract mathematical structures are, the more is the potential of their applicability to reality. My conception of the quality of mathematics came to be mediated by its power to be devoid of reality-derived meaning and at the same time its potential to be applied to different situations in the real world.

After completing the Bachelor's degree in mathematics and the Teaching Diploma in the teaching of mathematics, I decided to follow a Master's degree in mathematics at AUB, and luckily was granted a teaching assistantship. My experiences while studying for that degree did not seem to add to my concept of equity in mathematics education or to my conception of the nature of mathematics. However, during that period, I was initiated into the real world of teaching mathematics from two entry points: First, during my study for the Master's degree, I had to teach freshman mathematics courses as part of my assistantship, and second, I concurrently started to be a part-time secondary school mathematics teacher. Both teaching experiences reinforced my conception of the teaching of mathematics that I had formed, based on experiences with my former mathematics teachers and my experience during my undergraduate study at AUB. At the time I viewed math teaching as a delivery act which involved the presentation and explanation of mathematical concepts in a clear, correct, and systematic way. The teaching act normally ended with assessment, which constituted the basis for judging students: Those who did not meet the 'standard' for success were judged to be deficient in their abilities or in their background knowledge. I rarely thought that the emotional, social, economic, or family background could influence how students learned, what they learned, or how much they learned. In other words, for me, at that time, the learning of mathematics was the direct result of its teaching, and the success in learning mathematics was contingent on the skill of the teacher and ability and effort of the student. There was hardly any awareness, on my part, of the social, cultural, or emotional factors involved during the process of learning mathematics.

My university education at AUB came to a conclusion in 1968 with little, if any, awareness of issues of equity in education, let alone mathematics education. For me, at that time, the quality of mathematics learning was the degree to which the nature of mathematics as a study of structures was conveyed through its teaching. Little did I know that the new mathematics movement was being debated in the United States and that the essence of that movement was the emphasis on mathematical structure in curriculum and instruction, nor did I know that a new field called mathematics education was struggling to be born!

1.3 The Start of a Career in Mathematics Education

My career as a mathematics educator started when, upon graduation from AUB, I took the job of an assistant teacher training specialist in mathematics at the Institute of Education run jointly by UNRWA (United Nations Relief and Works Agency for Palestine Refugees in the Near East) and UNESCO. The Institute of Education provided long- and short-term in-service teacher education programs, including mathematics education, to teachers in Palestinian refugee camps in the West Bank and Gaza as well as in the refugee host countries (Lebanon, Jordan, and Syria). My job was to cooperate with the UNESCO mathematics education specialist to design and supervise the implementation of the mathematics education courses for mathematics teachers in all UNRWA schools. In the course of my job, I had to visit the UNRWA schools in the Palestinian camps regularly and conduct training sessions for teachers there.

My experiences in the UNRWA schools shook my long-held beliefs about equity. Here I came face to face with a human tragedy, where the Palestinian people in their totality were uprooted by force and intimidation from their homes in their country Palestine, to be accommodated in refugees camps with minimal provisions for survival. On the one hand, I had a chance to experience the glaring inequities evident in the daily life of the people in the camps as well as in the schools and to realize that these inequities were not the result of social injustice but human injustice. On the other hand, I also experienced the human compassion reflected in the tremendous efforts of UNRWA to provide subsistence and education via its schools, which were comparable to, and even better than, public schools in the Arab countries hosting the Palestinian refugees. Now that I reflect on that experience, I realize that education in the Palestinian camps was more meaningful to the people than any of the many countries I had the chance to know. However, I could not single out the inequities that related to mathematics education, since inequities in all aspects of their lives were so pervasive and so deep to the point that looking at those related to math education seemed to be a fruitless and non-consequential exercise.

My conception of what constituted mathematics education was also shaken by my experiences in UNRWA schools. I remember the frustrations I had in conveying the deep meaning of the mathematical ideas to the teachers to help them develop an advanced perspective of elementary mathematics. Teachers and students did not seem to see the relevance of mathematics to their lives. However, they saw the importance of mathematics for their advancement in school and for better opportunities for work and further education. I conjecture also that mathematics may have played a positive psychological role by providing children with a space to reason and contemplate, away from their harsh reality.

I learned two lessons from my work with the UNRWA Institute of Education. First, I had a reconstructed concept of equity in education in general, but not necessarily equity in mathematics education. However, this concept remained in my mind context-specific, namely, closely linked to the special situation of the Palestinian camps, and hence was not a universal concept applicable to all situations. Second, I learned that individuals hold different valuations and meanings of mathematics.

My work with UNRWA/UNESCO Institute of Education ended in 1971 when I accepted a fellowship to study for a PhD in mathematics education at the University of Wisconsin-Madison. The fellowship was part of a program aimed at building a capacity in science and mathematics education at the American University of Beirut in order to form a center for science and mathematics education there. At the time I accepted the offer, the Science and Mathematics Center had already been established and included four science educators who had completed the fellowship program at the University of Wisconsin-Madison but no mathematics educator.

My study at Madison-Wisconsin did not impact my beliefs and conceptions regarding equity and quality in mathematics education. However, I was initiated, for the first time, into research issues in mathematics education and research methods in social sciences. I also took graduate courses in the foundations of mathematics and was exposed to Godel's work, which seemed to push mathematics to its formalistic extreme. This reinforced the conception I held about mathematics as having no specific meaning in reality, which allows it to assume different 'meanings' and consequently renders it applicable to situations in all domains. This tension between the 'power' and 'meaning' in mathematics has since then dominated my conception of mathematics and its applications (Jurdak, 1999).

As an indication of the robustness of my beliefs regarding equity and quality of mathematics education, formed during earlier years, I give the example of my PhD dissertation. During my studies at Madison-Wisconsin, I came to learn about the debate that dominated mathematics education in the USA during the sixties and the central role of mathematical structure in that debate (see Chapter 2). This seemed to validate and reinforce my already held beliefs about the nature of mathematics and the central role of mathematical structure in organizing and delivering the mathematics curriculum to the extent that I chose this title for my PhD dissertation 'The Effects of Emphasizing Mathematical Structural Properties in Teaching and of Reflective Intelligence on Four Selected Criteria' (Jurdak, 1973). This topic was not unusual at the time, but the context in which the dissertation study was carried out was. The teaching experiment for the dissertation was conducted in Lebanon in two school systems which accommodated students with diametrically opposite socioeconomic and even cultural backgrounds: One was the UNRWA school system which served the children of the Palestinian refugees in Lebanon and the second was the most exclusive school in the country. However, the dissertation did not try, in any way, to explain the learning of students in terms of their socioeconomic or cultural backgrounds but focused on the effect of teaching mathematical structure on mathematics learning. The study as conducted did not take note of the social context and assumed it could have been conducted anywhere with the same methods and probably with the same conclusions. Although it looks odd, and perhaps extreme, the study reflected the kind of thinking regarding the social aspect of mathematics education held at the time.

I finished my PhD in 1973 and joined the Department of Education and the Science and Mathematics Education Center (SMEC) at AUB. As happens often, I started my career there by developing the courses for the Master's degree in mathematics education. As a young assistant professor, I was inspired, in this foundational phase, by my professors and their courses at the University of Wisconsin- Madison. My teaching at AUB and my supervision of MA theses had little impact on my belief system regarding equity and quality in mathematics education. I was still under the spell of mathematical structure. However, in my first independent research project, I shifted a little towards logical inference and its relation to language. Attempting to publish a paper on my project in a scholarly journal was a remarkably daring feat. For some reason, the journal of *Educational Studies in Mathematics* (ESM) attracted my attention because it dealt with topics similar to my project. The editor of ESM was Freudenthal himself, one of the early fathers of mathematics education. He was the the founder, editor, and the single unrefutable referee of ESM. Frankly, I was not intimidated to send the manuscript to ESM simply because I was not aware then of the weight and temper of Freudenthal. To my great surprise, I received a letter from Freudenthal responding to my submission in strong and unquestionable authority to tell me that, unlike some of the 'rubbish' he received, there may be something good in my manuscript but I needed to work on it. I did revise the manuscript and it was eventually published (Jurdak, 1977).

My first experience with publishing in international mathematics education journals taught me a few lessons. The first lesson was that the acceptance of manuscripts for publication in international journals was fair and equitable. Admittedly the acceptance of my paper at that time was not based on a blind review; however, only a visionary arching authority like Freudenthal could accept a manuscript on the basis of what he solely considered merit in it, without regard to the fact that I was a first-time unknown author from a small developing country. This experience encouraged me to continue my career as a mathematics education researcher. The second lesson was that I started to learn the 'trade' of publishing in international journals and to realize that the community of mathematics education researchers, at least at that time, was more concerned with defining the identity of the emerging field of mathematics education and establishing its scientific validity than with the needs of the mathematics education community of practitioners.

An experience which had a lasting impact on my conception of equity and quality in mathematics education was my involvement in several curriculum development projects in some Arab countries. This brought me face to face with equity and quality issues in the actual world of policy makers, schools, teachers, and students. Through institutional arrangement between the American University of Beirut and some Arab ministries of education, the Science and Mathematics Education Center (SMEC) was charged with implementing science and mathematics curriculum development in some Arab countries. I assumed the leadership role in the mathematics education of these projects. I shall cite the examples of my curriculum development experiences in Saudi Arabia and Sudan to illustrate how my conceptions of equity and quality were mediated by my experiences in two socioeconomically and culturally different countries. Saudi Arabia was an oil-rich kingdom with vast financial resources and very ambitious plans for social development but within a strict interpretation of Islam. The Sudan, on the other hand, was a poor vast agrarian republic with limited financial resources to meet its development needs. Culturally, Saudi Arabia is an ethnically, linguistically, and religiously homogeneous Moslem society, whereas Sudan is an ethnically, linguistically, and religiously diverse society. The education system in Saudi Arabia grew out of religious community schools to become a vast public education system whose schools were equipped with modern facilities and mostly expatriate teachers from other Arab countries, mainly from Egypt; whereas, the education system in Sudan was modeled in its educational approach after that of Britain, which had ruled the country before the fifties. The Sudanese schools lacked in facilities and equipment but were in good supply of well-prepared Sudanese teachers. Unlike Saudi Arabia, Sudan had a unique tradition in teacher education. In the 1930s, Griffiths, one of HMI inspectors of education, decided to establish an institution to prepare teachers for rural areas and set up an institute of education, calling it Bakht-Al-Rida after the name of the nearest little village. There he built a campus with minimal facilities similar to what one would expect in the rural areas of Sudan. The recruited student teachers were required to live on campus and lead a combined life of work and education in this minimalist environment. The student teachers as a group were expected to develop, test, and debate the school curriculum, lesson by lesson. Bakht-Al-Rida became known in East Africa and its model attracted the attention of the United Nations organization which looked up to it as a relevant and successful model for rural education. Griffiths documented the establishment of Bakht-Al-Rida and his experiences there in a book, now out of print, under the title *An Experiment in Education* (Griffiths, 1953).

As a result of my work in the curriculum projects in Saudi Arabia and Sudan, my conception of mathematics education was challenged by my experiences. For about five years in the mid-seventies, our team had the chance to work with teams of local mathematics educators and to visit schools and meet with teachers in both Saudi Arabia and Sudan. The socioeconomic and cultural contrast between Saudi Arabia and Sudan sharpened my awareness of the complexity of how and to what extent socioeconomic and cultural contexts mediate student mathematics learning.

Prior to my engagement in these curriculum development projects I tended to view the school as a production system and thus, by improving the quantity and quality of the input (facilities, textbooks, equipment, human resources..) and the quality and efficiency of the processes, the output of the system would most likely improve. This view was challenged by the contrast in math education between Saudi Arabia and Sudan. More than Sudan, Saudi Arabia could afford to provide for its students more and better input for mathematics learning including experienced expatriate teachers. For example, the school buildings were well-designed with proper facilities; whereas in Sudan, school buildings were old houses, with not enough space to seat children. The mathematics textbooks (the ones we prepared at SMEC) for Saudi Arabia were comparable in content and production to the best books produced in the USA, whereas the mathematics textbooks in Sudan were old and poorly produced and were insufficient for the needs of the students. According to the production system, one would expect that the learning outcomes would be better in Saudi Arabia than in Sudan. This was not actually the case and in fact, my impression was that the learning of mathematics was more meaningful and enjoyable to Sudanese than to Saudi children. At that time it was not easy to resolve this discrepancy, but in a hindsight I attribute it to my view of an educational system as a production system, which did not account for the social-cultural context of learning mathematics. From my *perspective now*, I would conjecture that the discrepancy may be explained in terms of social-cultural factors. For example, could it be that the tradition of preparing teachers in a rural environment at Bakht-Al-Rida in the Sudan had equipped the teachers with the attitudes and skills to engage their students in more relevant learning? Could it be that the scarcity of textbooks and their low-quality production might have pushed the teachers to focus on mental computational strategies or to resort to their environment for resources for teaching and learning? Were the textbooks we prepared for the Saudi students not culturally relevant? Was the incompatibility between the home habitus and school more in Saudi Arabia than in Sudan? If these questions had ever crossed my mind at the time, they would not have been perceived by me as legitimate mathematics education *research questions* then.

I emerged from the seventies with a double identity: The identity of a mathematics education researcher and that of a mathematics educator. There was a sharp demarcation between the two identities. The researcher identity made me conform, without much regard to implications of my research to practice, to the standards set by the community of mathematics education researchers, which was attempting to define the identity of mathematics education and establish its scientific validity. On the other hand, the mathematics educator identity pushed me to use my expertise in the field to give judgements and recommendations to policy makers and practitioners with little regard to research findings. Like mathematics education in the seventies, I was searching for my professional identity. It took another ten years for the two identities to be integrated!

1.4 The Nineteen Eighties: The Beginning of the Social Turn

Although my awareness of the social and cultural aspects of mathematics education was sharpened in the seventies, it remained at the level of experience and did not reach the level of scholarly discourse. My first experience with participating in a scholarly discourse on the topic of goals as related to social and cultural needs was in the UNESCO Meeting of Experts on Goals for Mathematics Education: Mathematics Teaching and the needs of Society (Paris, 19–23, May 1980). The Meeting assembled a group of 12 representatives of UNESCO Member States and representatives of the International Commission on Mathematical Instruction (ICMI), the World Federation of the Teaching Profession, and of the International Baccalaureat. For the first time, I had the chance to participate in scholarly discourse on topics that had not been discussed before in scholarly conferences and journals. Such topics included: Goals as a reflection of the needs of society, the learner, and the requirements of production; goals of mathematics for rural development; links with commerce and industry (Morris, 1981). My contribution was a paper co-authored with Ed Jacobsen 'The evolution of mathematics curricula in the Arab States' (Jurdak and Jacobsen, 1981). The UNESCO Paris meeting in terms of its participants, topics, and emphasis on the role of mathematics in serving the needs of society provided a validation for the scholarly legitimacy of my beliefs, gained through my experiences, regarding the social and cultural aspects of mathematics education. On the other hand it broadened my narrow conception of mathematics education as a purely mathematical act to one that had social and cultural determinants. The Paris Meeting was a small and intimate professional gathering which combined the lively and non-formal discussions inside the conference room and the discussions over dinners in Paris restaurants. It was a great chance for me to interact professionally and personally with colleagues of similar interests. Because of the topics, format, size, and venue, I formed lasting friendships with many colleagues whose friendship I renewed during ICME's, especially, Mogens Niss, Ubiratan D'Ambrosio, and Ed Jacobsen.

In the same year, I attended my first ICME in Berkeley, USA, and what a contrast ICME was compared to our meeting in Paris! From my perspective as a first-time participant from a small developing country, ICME was overwhelmingly big, impersonal, and intimidating in its structure and participants, and this reflected the power structure between developed and developing countries. ICME was my first experience of inequitable participation in international mathematics education activities.

During the early eighties, my beliefs about the social and cultural contexts of mathematics education, remained at the level of convictions rather than guiding research principles. So I continued my research along the same line as in the seventies. My research was still dominated by the idea of mathematical structures, but toned down to link it to classroom problem solving and activities. The following two studies were typical of my research concerns in the eighties: The facilitating effect of structured games in mathematics (Jurdak and Ibrahim, 1982) and the role of sequence and context in structurally-related problems (Jurdak, 1985).

One important event in the development of my conception of the social and cultural aspects of mathematics education was ICME 6 in Budapest, Hungary in 1988. The Congress devoted its entire fifth day to the topic 'Mathematics, Education, and Society'. On the fifth day, I gave a presentation entitled 'Religion and Language as Cultural Carriers and Barriers in Mathematics Education' (Jurdak, 1989), in which I examined the way ideology, particularly religion, and language of instruction (foreign or native) were cultural carriers in mathematics education and may act as barriers to learning mathematics in conflict situations. From the response I received, I felt I had struck some novel and thought-provoking ideas by suggesting that religion and language may impact mathematics education in conflict situations.

In hindsight, I can now retrace the roots of these ideas to the historicity of my experiences. First, the Paris meeting had helped me re-orient my conception of the relationship between mathematics education, society, and culture; second, during the eighties I experienced the violent conflicts in Lebanon, which one could partially relate to conflicting cultural identities, involving religion and language; third, my curriculum development experiences in Saudi Arabia, Sudan, and Lebanon helped me realize how ideologies which were thought to be too far removed from mathematics, often perceived as culture-free and hence immune to cultural conflicts, impact mathematics education in a significant way.

By the end of eighties, I emerged with a more coherent professional identity by reconciling the two identities of mathematics educator and researcher. In Budapest, I was able to pull together my experiences in curriculum development and my conception of the social and cultural aspects of mathematics education. At that time, my beliefs shifted from a neutral attitude towards the social and cultural aspects of mathematics education to a more politically-oriented critical attitude towards inequities in mathematics education resulting from social and cultural conflicts. The experiences of the eighties sharpened my awareness of inequities in mathematics education.

1.5 The Nineteen Nineties: Problem Solving in School and Outside

The momentum of the late eighties in the development of my conceptions of social and cultural conflicts and inequities in mathematics education seemed to thrust my thinking towards more global conceptions of inequity and quality in mathematics education. These conceptions were reflected in my lecture entitled 'Mathematics Education in the Global Village: The Wedge and the Filter' (Jurdak, 1992) presented at ICME 7 in Laval, Canada. In this paper I argued that mathematics education does not act only as a filter to scientific and professional fields but also as a wedge among mathematics education communities in developing and developed countries. I also argued that the divide in the quality of mathematics education between developing and developed countries is not likely to shrink and that will probably impose a separate development (apartheid) model in mathematics education in the developing countries. The link between equity and quality started to be formed at that time.

The ICME 7 lecture seemed to me as far as I could go in that direction because, up to then, my statements regarding equity and quality at the international level were ideological in nature, or at best hypotheses which required, for their support, evidence from an international mathematics education database, not available at the time. This necessitated a new direction on my part in order to be able to test some of these ideas in the real world of schools. So I decided to shift my interest from the macro to the micro and from the global ideology of mathematics education to mathematics pedagogy in schools. Still I was eager to incorporate in this new direction the dialectical relationship between mathematics in the school and the social context outside.

Towards the middle of the nineties, I chose problem solving as a focus to explore the tension between mathematics in the classroom and its application in the real world. With the help of my students, I started a series of studies to explore problem solving in the school and outside it. The first of those studies compared and contrasted the computational strategies used by young vendors in the streets of Beirut in the course of their daily work and those used by regular students (Jurdak and Shahin, 1999). There was clear evidence of more effective use of logico-mathematical properties in transactions by the vendors than in word problems or computational exercises by the students. We used a variety of theoretical frameworks, including cognitive theories, to explain these results; however, none explained the results to our satisfaction. The results of this study blurred my conception of quality and equity in mathematics education and begged the following question: How could a less advantaged vendor engage in relatively high level mathematical processes, but on the other hand, have no opportunity to continue further education, whereas an advantaged student in a school was less able to engage in high level computational strategies, and yet have all the opportunities to continue further education?

The second study entitled 'Problem Solving Activity in the Workplace and the School: The Case of Constructing Solids' (Jurdak and Shahin, 2001) documented, compared, and analyzed the nature of spatial reasoning, while constructing solids, with given specifications, from plane surfaces done by practitioners (a plumber) in the workplace, and students in the school setting . The differences between the approaches and solutions of students and plumber were very obvious and our search for a theoretical model which could explain such differences led us to the activity theory (Leont'ev, 1981). A central assertion of activity theory is that our knowledge of the world is mediated by our interaction with it, and thus, human behavior and thinking occur within meaningful contexts as people conduct purposeful goal-directed activities. Moreover, learning takes place in a community of practice and is mediated by the artifacts used by that community. For me activity theory provided the missing link between 'doing and thinking' and more importantly between the roles of individual and community in human activity. Activity theory provided a satisfactory explanation of the differences between the context of practice and the context of school. The differences between the two contexts is in fact due to the seemingly similar but really different goal structures. In the school context, the goal of the problem solving activity is to solve this problem for an academic purpose which is concretely embodied in getting credit (score or grade) for the solution. To achieve that goal, students use artifacts that are deemed appropriate for that purpose; i.e. thinking, mathematical language, writing on paper. On the other hand, the practitioner's goal is to manufacture certain products with a set of specifications. The manufacturing might require, among other things, some use of mathematical tools. The practitioner resorts to artifacts (physical tools, measurement, language, advice from manuals or others) to achieve that goal. The goal is achieved if the product is made according to specifications. So the student and the practitioner have in fact different activity structures. Even after this study, the paradoxical relationship between equity and quality in mathematics education remained as blurred as before.

The nineties witnessed my adoption of a macro rather than a micro perspective regarding the relation of mathematics education to social and cultural contexts by refocusing my research activities on contrasting problem solving inside and outside school. Towards the end of the nineties I acquired the theoretical framework of activity theory which helped me better understand problem solving in school and in practice. This provided me with a sociocultural lens to look at differences between the learning of mathematics in school and applying it in the real world. The tension in the relationship between quality and equity in mathematics education had yet to be resolved in my mind.

1.6 The Present: Reflecting on the Past and Looking Ahead

The first decade of the twenty-first century was an opportunity for me to consolidate my ideas regarding equity and quality in mathematics education. First, I extended my work on problem solving in and outside school by focusing on the perspective of high school students on problem solving inside and outside the school (Jurdak, 2006a). In this study we contrasted, theoretically and empirically, problem solving in three contexts, the real world, the situated school context, and the non-situated school context. The results indicated that there were fundamental identifiable differences in problem solving activity in the three contexts. The construct of the activity system, which was used in this study as an analytical framework, proved to be a powerful construct for organizing my emerging new conceptions of the relationships among mathematics, society, and culture. The activity system seemed to me to be a powerful socialcultural theoretical framework for studying equity in quality in institutional mathematics education as a collective activity in different contexts (see Chapter 3).

My first experience with TIMSS 2003 (Trends in International Mathematics and Science Study) data was when I was commissioned by UNESCO Regional Office for Arab States to use the data for the eight Arab countries, which participated in TIMSS 2003 to conduct a study on the impact of student, teacher, and school factors on achievement in mathematics and science (Jurdak, 2006b). To achieve the purpose of the study, I defined the impact of a particular factor on mathematics achievement to be the proportion of variance accounted for by that factor. In comparing the impact of the student, teacher, and school factors on mathematics achievement, within and across the eight countries, it became apparent to me that, in fact, the differential impact of these factors on mathematics achievement was actually a measure of inequity in mathematics achievement. The UNESCO study suggested that the TIMSS background questionnaire data may be used to study equity issues within a country (comparison of the impact of factors in a country) and across countries (comparison of the impact of a factor across countries). The UNESCO study inspired the use of TIMSS database to compare inequities across countries and provided a dry run of the approach adopted in Part II of this book.

The book concept on the subject of equity in quality was triggered by the the activity system and the UNESCO study. However, the book concept was an opportunity to reflect on my own experiences and analyze the sociocultural research in mathematics education from the perspective of equity and quality and to use data from a vast international comparative study such as TIMSS to test some of the many claims made in this area. Following the approval of the book proposal by Springer, two more events helped develop the ideas presented in this book. The first event was the invitation to give a plenary session in the fifth conference of Mathematics and Society (MES 5) and my lecture there was entitled 'Towards a Theoretical Framework for Equity in Quality' which formed the basis for Chapter 3 of this book. The second event was the invitation I received from ICME 11 to be on a plenary Panel on 'equal access to quality mathematics education' and my presentation was entitled 'Equity in Quality in Math Education – A Global Perspective' which formed the basis of Chapter 11 of this book. These two events served as landmarks in my journey towards equity in quality.

In this book I tell three versions of the story of equity and quality: The first is mine, the second is the story of equity and quality in mathematics education, and the third is the story of educational equity and quality in general (Chapter 2). These stories converge and diverge at many points. My story seems to be closer to that of mathematics education, simply because I and mathematics education, as a field of study, are about the same age. I hope the reader will enjoy this book as much as I enjoyed the journey to get to it.

Historical Evolution of Equity and Quality in Education and in Math Education

This chapter will present a comparative historical account of the evolution of issues of quality and equity in mathematics education and education in general. The historical account will be limited to the second half of the twentieth century when issues had started to be debated at the scholarly and policy levels. It will also be at the macro level focusing on international reports and literature.

The issues of educational equity and quality will be traced historically with reference to the United Nations treaties and declarations pertaining to the right to education. The issues of equity and quality in mathematics education will be traced with reference to three types of publications of historical value in mathematics education: Landmark scholarly publications, reports written by authorities in the field, and the activities of the International Commission on Mathematics Instruction (ICMI), including the International Conferences on Mathematics Education (ICME conferences) and ICMI studies.

2.1 The Evolution of Educational Equity and Quality

2.1.1 The Fifties and Sixties

In 1948, the United Nations made a declaration about the nature and extent of human rights amongst which was the right to education for all people. It was declared that elementary education would be free and compulsory and that the higher levels of education would be accessible to all on the basis of merit (United Nations, 1948, Article 26). The UN declaration of human rights was transformed into action at the international level through the use of treaties as instruments to secure human rights observance. Between 1976 and 1990 a series of international covenants and conventions were developed to provide a comprehensive legal basis for the measures required to protect and deliver human rights.

M. Jurdak, *Toward Equity in Quality in Mathematics Education*,
DOI 10.1007/978-1-4419-0558-1_2,
© Springer Science+Business Media, LLC 2009

The earliest two of those treaties which affected education were the International Covenant on Civil and Political Rights (ICCPR) (United Nations, 1966a) and the International Covenant on Economic, Social and Cultural Rights (ICESCR) (United Nations, 1966b), which together with the Universal Declaration of Human Rights (United Nations, 1948), have been proclaimed by the United Nations to constitute the International Bill of Human Rights. All of these treaties reaffirmed the right to compulsory and free primary education, and nondiscrimination in educational provisions first set out in the 1948 Declaration.

According to the UN regulations, treaties are expected to be ratified by the member states, and when this happens, the treaty becomes legally binding for the state. Each treaty requires the government's periodic self assessment of its compliance and a binding reporting procedure to the UN.

2.1.2 The Seventies

The Universal Primary Education (UPE) was a moving target. The educational commitments made in the Universal Declaration of Human Rights have also been reaffirmed on many occasions by UNESCO actions. UNESCO established 1980 as a target date for the achievement of universal primary education (UPE) in most of the developing regions of the world. However, this target was not achieved.

One of the earliest of UNESCO's visions of the quality of education appeared in the report of the International Commission on the Development of Education which was chaired by Edgar Faure (Faure et al., 1972). The vision of this landmark report introduced the concept of lifelong education as a right for every individual and reaffirmed that universal basic education, in a variety of forms, depending on possibilities and needs, should be the top priority for educational policies in the 1970s.

2.1.3 The Eighties

The eighties did not witness significant progress either in achieving the target of universal primary education or in bringing forward new conceptualizations of educational quality. It was a decade for reaffirming the original recommendations of the Bill of Human Rights regarding the right of the child to free and compulsory primary education without discrimination and the right of accessibility to higher levels of education for all on the basis of merit.

2.1.4 The Nineties

By 1990, however, there was still a long way to go, and the World Conference on Education for All, was held that year in Jomtien (Thailand). In addition to restating the UPE goal for achievement by the year 2000, the Jomtien Conference (UUNESCO, 1990) set out an 'expanded vision for education' which stipulated that beside expanding access to education, education should contribute fully to individual and societal development through focus on learning, relevance, and quality of education as prerequisites for achieving the fundamental goal of equity. Although great progress had been made in most regions, the target, again, was not fully realized by all countries. Accordingly, in 2000, the Millennium Declaration (United Nations, 2000) reaffirmed that children everywhere, boys and girls alike, should be able to complete a full course of primary schooling, but did not go beyond that.

In the mid nineties another landmark report by the International Commission of Education for the twenty-first century, chaired by Jacques Delors came with a report titled 'Learning: The Treasure Within' (Delores et al., 1996). The report identified the goal of education as based on its ability to provide learning to know, learning to do, learning to live together, and learning to be.

Up till the Millennium Declaration, the UN treaties and declarations focused on providing Universal Primary Education (UPE) without discrimination but they were almost silent on the quality of education. The Jomtien World Declaration on Education for All (UNESCO, 1990) was more of a vision than a plan of action. In 2000, The Dakar Framework for Action (UNESCO, 2000) set out an ambitious and comprehensive agenda to be achieved by 2015.

2.1.5 The First Decade of the Twenty-First Century

In 2000, The Dakar Framework for Action (UNESCO, 2000) specified the following goals:

1. Expanding and improving comprehensive early childhood care and education, especially for the most vulnerable and disadvantaged children.
2. Ensuring that by 2015, all children, particularly girls, children in difficult circumstances and those belonging to ethnic minorities, have access to complete free and compulsory primary education of good quality.
3. Ensuring that the learning needs of all young people and adults are met through equitable access to appropriate learning and life skills programmes.
4. Achieving a 50% improvement in the level of adult literacy by 2015, especially for women,and equitable access to basic and continuing education for all adults.
5. Eliminating gender disparities in primary and secondary education by 2005, and achieving gender equality in education by 2015, ensuring girls' full and equal access to and achievement in basic education of good quality.
6. Improving all aspects of the quality of education and ensuring excellence of all so that recognized and measurable learning outcomes are achieved by all, especially in literacy, numeracy and essential life skills.

The Dakar Framework was a significant landmark in the international declarations regarding educational equity and quality. First, it was the first time in the declarations of the UN bodies that equity and quality of education were put together as goals of education within a framework of action and within a specific time line. It brought forward the argument that the achievement of the moving target of universal participation in education may be dependent on the quality of education provided. It underscored that the quality of teaching and student learning may have an impact on how long students stay in school and how punctual they are in their attendance and participation in learning. Parents, on the other hand, are more likely to send their children to school if they perceive that the quality and relevance of their children's education justify the investment they are making. Also the quality goal specifies that the quality of all aspects of education should be ensured, and that measurable learning outcomes be achieved by all, especially in literacy, numeracy, and essential life skills (goal 6). Moreover, the Dakar Framework is the most comprehensive in all UN declarations regarding education in that it extends the agenda beyond achieving universal participation in education in two directions; improving early childhood education (goal 1), and providing for adult continuing education through ensuring that the needs of all young people and adults are met through equitable access to appropriate learning and life skills programmes (goal 3 and 4).

In summary, the pattern of evolution of the concepts of equity and quality seem to have been dominated by equity in the decades that followed the founding of the United Nations. The concept of quality in education was put forward as an international concern only towards the turn of the last century. New daring visions of educational quality were formulated in the seventies and nineties but were not translated into action then. The Dakar Framework marks the birth of the concept of equity in quality in education, a concept advocated for mathematics education in this book. The Dakar Framework underlined the interdependence between equity and quality and set out an agenda based on the assumption that educational processes and outcomes are qualitative in nature and that the number of children who participate in education is not a substitute for the quality of their education.

2.2 The Evolution of Equity and Quality in Mathematics Education Literature

2.2.1 The Fifties and Sixties

Unlike the evolution of educational equity and quality, the evolution of equity and quality in mathematics education was dominated by quality issues between 1950 and 1980. The evolution of the concepts of equity and quality in mathematics education in the second half of the last century will be traced by referring to three categories of publications of historical value in this regard: Landmark scholarly publications, reports written by authorities in the field, and the activities of the International Commission on Mathematics Instruction (ICMI).

The 1950s witnessed the 'new mathematics' movement in the United States of America and later in other developed countries. The motivation and the characteristics of this movement have been documented in many studies (Begle, 1970; ICMI, 1979; Morris, 1980). The issues debated in this period were almost exclusively related to the improvement of the quality of mathematics education. In the area of the goals, the debate focused on rationalizing new reasons for more expanded mathematical education by broadening its goals to encompass all aspects of mathematical literacy (Niss, 1996). The rationalizations for improving the quality of these goals were varied and included economic competitiveness, the development of mathematical knowledge, the role of mathematics in the sciences, the needs of the modern workplace, and the needs of the information age.

The improvement of mathematical content and its organization in the curriculum were the paramount concern of that era. One of the publications which captured the ethos of the new mathematics movement was the sixty-ninth yearbook on 'Mathematics Education' published by the National Society for the Study of Education (NSSE) (1970). The significance of this yearbook is that the NSSE publishes a yearbook on an educational subject, if its board of directors senses that there is a turning point in the development of that subject. Before the NSSE 1970 yearbook, the last yearbook that the NSSE published on mathematics was in 1951 on The Teaching of Arithmetic (NSSE, 1951). In the preface of the NSSE (1970) yearbook, the editor of the series wrote:

> "In 1966, the Board of Directors of the National Society sensing that the shock wave of the radical changes in pre-college mathematics of the past decade or so was subsiding, concluded that it would be appropriate to prepare a clear account of the changes that had occurred and to examine the implications of those changes for mathematics teaching in the near future" (p. vii)

In the introduction of the yearbook, Edward Begle (1966), the editor of the yearbook wrote:

> "Not quite two decades have elapsed since the appearance of the last NSSE yearbook on mathematics education. During that period a revolution in school mathematics has taken place... This revolution in school mathematics was, in a sense, a byproduct of a revolution in mathematics itself." (p. 1)

In support of the innovation in mathematics curricula, Wilder (1970) presented arguments which were typical of the many arguments given in that era. One argument was that mathematical knowledge was growing rapidly both in its basic and applied aspects. Consequently, it was expected that more topics considered to be university subjects would be provided at the high school level and some topics at the high school level would be moved to the primary level. A second argument was that this transfer of topics could not be done by adding new topics to the existing ones in the curriculum, so to accomplish this transfer, a new organization of the curriculum had to be introduced. This organization was based on mathematics as a study of structures - known as the 'economy principle' - since studying a mathematical structure would save instructional time because many mathematical topics could be regarded as examples of that structure. The third argument was that such a curriculum would not only bring up-to-date mathematical knowledge but will also enable students to exercise mathematical ways of thought.

The new mathematics movement was reinforced by a psychology of learning that was aligned with the nature of the new mathematics education. It was Bruner who was able to capture the spirit of the movement and provide a framework for a cognitive theory. In his book, *The Process of Education*, Bruner (1960) presents four themes, two of which capture and reinforce the spirit of the new mathematics movement: The importance of structure and readiness for learning. In the theme of structure, Bruner states that:

> "grasping the structure of a subject is understanding it in a way that permits many other things to be related to it meaningfully. To learn structure, in short is to learn how thing are related" (p. 7)

He further argues that understanding fundamentals makes a subject more comprehensible, ensures more effective retention, promotes the transfer of learning, and narrows the gap between 'elementary' knowledge and 'advanced' knowledge. Bruner's ideas regarding the structure of a subject, reinforced the basic assumptions made by the new mathematics movement about the importance of organizing mathematics curricula around mathematical structures.

On the theme of readiness for learning, Bruner makes the startling statement that:

> "we begin with the hypothesis that any subject can be taught effectively in some intellectually honest form to any child at any stage of development." (p. 33)

This view of readiness for learning rationalized (or motivated) the proposals of the new mathematics movement to push down advanced topics in mathematics from the university level to secondary and even primary levels. Seemingly, Bruner's statement on readiness for learning implied a strong position on equality, by affirming the equality of humans in their potential to learn; however, it was not a statement about equity from a social justice perspective.

The pre-occupation with the quality of mathematics education rather than the equity in access to it was also evident in the developing countries. One example in the developing countries was the UNESCO Mathematics Project for the Arab States (UMPAS) (UNESCO, 1969) which was typical of the effort of the international community to 'transfer' the experience of the developed countries to developing countries. As the 'revolution' of the new mathematics movement was about to fade away in western countries, UNESCO decided to sponsor a mathematics project in the Arab countries to improve the quality of mathematics education, in harmony with similar projects undertaken in the developed countries. UNESCO brought together many of the prominent leaders of the new mathematics movement to put together a vision and a mathematics curriculum at the secondary level. The rationalization given for such a vision echoed the one given in the United States in the 1950s as evidenced by the following statement that appeared in an early project document (UNESCO, 1966):

> "Modernization means that the teaching of mathematics is based on a general attitude quite different from the one in traditional teaching. It proceeds, using the notion of set theory as a basis, to build up a more unified construction, structured by homogeneous ideas. Mathematics must be taught by stressing, at the appropriate time, the fundamental structures that occur in several branches of mathematics, both as means and ends" (Appendix II)

UMPAS was meant to be a starting point for a sustainable development of mathematics education in the Arab countries. However, because of its excesses and its over-emphasis on abstract concepts and mathematical structure, the long term impact of UMPAS withered away in a few years.

2.2.2 The Seventies

The seventies were years of questioning of and doubt in the promises of the new mathematics era. One extreme reaction to that was to return to the basics, that is, to emphasize skills through drill work without consideration for building understanding and to do away with the abstraction and the excessive emphasis on mathematical processes and mathematical topics that do not have direct application in school or in life.

2.2.3 The Eighties

The early eighties witnessed a shift towards connecting mathematics education to academic and adult life needs, societal needs, and technological needs. Thus, the link with society became one important attribute in the quality of mathematics education. Although individual differences were recognized in this respect, they were not seen as equity issues that should be addressed from a social responsibility perspective. We present two examples to illustrate the shift in the goals of math towards being more inclusive of individual and societal needs.

The first example comes from a UNESCO publication (Morris, 1981) based on papers presented in a meeting which brought together 14 math educators representing different parts of the world and relevant international organizations to debate and review the question of goals of mathematics education. Perhaps the best way to convey the spirit of the meeting and the publication that followed is to list some of the titles of the papers presented and debated:

1. Goals as a reflection of the needs of society
2. Goals as a reflection of the needs of the learner
3. Goals as a reflection of the needs of the requirements of production
4. Goals of mathematics for rural development
5. Links with commerce and industry
6. Educational objectives for mathematics compatible with its development as a discipline
7. New goals for old: An analysis of reactions to recent reforms in several countries
8. The NCTM PRISM project: An attempt to make curriculum change more rational and systematic
9. The evolution of mathematics curricula in the Arab countries
10. Goals of the mathematics curriculum in British Columbia: Intended, implemented and realized.

The meeting, with its participants and topics and its emphasis on the role of mathematics in serving the different needs of the individual in school and adult life, the society, and the discipline, represented a shift from the new mathematics fundamental goals of understanding the nature of mathematics.

Another significant example that illustrates the shift in the goals of mathematics education towards more responsiveness to the needs of the individual and society was the Cockcroft Report entitled 'Mathematics Counts' (Committee of Inquiry into the Teaching of Mathematics in Schools, 1982). This committee was set by the government to consider and make recommendations regarding teaching math in primary schools in England and Wales, with particular regard to the mathematics required for further and higher education, employment and adult life. Committee membership included research mathematicians, mathematics educators, higher education professors and administrators, school teachers and administrators, representatives of industry and business, and representatives of the educational authorities. The committee worked for four years on its mission and submitted in 1982 a comprehensive report which came to be known as the Cockcroft Report after its chair W.H. Cockcroft.

The Cockcroft Report was a landmark in the history of mathematics education in the second half of the last century because of its impact on mathematics education, not only in England and Wales but in the rest of world. This is because it legitimized and transformed earlier ideas and visions into action plans as to how to render mathematics to count by re-orienting it to serve the needs of individuals (as learners and adults) in school, in employment, and in further and higher education.

2.2.4 The Nineties

The nineties of the last century witnessed the emergence of the concept of equal access to quality mathematics. This was heralded by an important report prepared by two boards, namely the Board on Mathematical Sciences and Mathematical Sciences Education Board (1989). The report was entitled 'Everybody Counts', which in comparison to the Cockcroft Report (Mathematics Counts), reflected, intentionally or unintentionally, the change towards more inclusive goals of mathematics education. Though *Everybody Counts* makes similar arguments regarding the importance of the role of mathematics in serving the needs of students' adult life in terms of employment and further education, it does however bring into focus three issues. First, it broadens mathematical literacy to be in line with the requirements of the information age. Second, it underlines the importance of mathematics for the economy and recommends doing away with the historically dominant idea of having a two-tier mathematical literacy, one for the masses and one for college bound students. Third, and most importantly, it declares explicitly that the quality of mathematics education is not achieved if equal participation in mathematics education is not provided: 'It is vitally important for society that *all* citizens benefit equally from high-quality mathematics education' p. 7.

Two curriculum projects which have had a far-reaching impact worldwide demonstrate the growing concern in the nineties regarding increasing the weight given to equal access to quality mathematics education: The National Curriculum in the United Kingdom and the National Council of Teachers of Mathematics (NCTM) in the USA. The National Curriculum included equal access to quality mathematics education among its aims. One of the aims in Stages 1 and 2 is 'The school curriculum should aim to provide opportunities for all pupils to learn and to achieve' (Qualifications and Curriculum Authority (QCA),1999). Also the National Curriculum included the following aim in Stages 3 and 4: 'The curriculum should enable all young people to become: Successful learners, who enjoy learning, make progress and achieve; confident individuals who are able to live safe, healthy and fulfilling lives; responsible citizens who make a positive contribution to society' (Qualifications and Curriculum Authority (QCA), 2007). In its project Standards 2000, the NCTM dedicated one out of its six principles to equity: 'Excellence in mathematics education requires equity-high expectations and strong support for all students' (NCTM, 2000). It is worth observing that the issue of equity did not come up in the NCTM Standards of 1989.

2.3 The Evolution of Equity and Quality in Mathematics Education in ICMI and PME Activities

We shall survey two types of ICMI (International Commission on Mathematics Instruction) activities: ICMI Studies and the International Congresses of Mathematics Education (ICME).

2.3.1 ICMI Studies

In the the past 17 years, ICMI studies mainly addressed issues related to the quality of mathematics education, with the exception of the following two studies which have relevance to equity issues in mathematics education:

- Gender and mathematics education, published under the title 'Towards Gender Equity in Mathematics Education' (Hanna, 1996)
- Mathematics education in different cultural traditions: a comparative study of east asia and the west (Leung et al., 2006)

2.3.2 The ICME Congresses

The main activities of ICME congresses from 1968 to 2008 were surveyed for their coverage of and relevance to equity issues in mathematics education. The activities surveyed were: Plenary sessions, non-plenary lectures, and conference groups (according to the different terminologies used: working groups, topic groups, discussion groups). The sources of information were: (1) The official programs of ICME congresses which I attended and and whose programs I have in my personal files (ICME 4 and ICME 6–11); (2) an ICMI web site (Furinghetti and Giacardi, 2008) for the remaining ICME congresses. The activities that pertain to equity in the remaining ICME congresses are listed in Figure 2.1 (1968–1988), Figure 2.2 (1992–2000), and Figure 2.3 (2004–2008). The results may be summarized as follows:

- The majority of ICME congresses focused on aspects of quality of mathematics education
- Each of the ICME congresses had at least one plenary lecture that pertained to equity issues except ICME congresses 1, 7, 8, and 9
- ICME 6 was a turning point as far as emphasis on social issues. In the ICME congresses that followed ICME 6, the number of lectures that pertained to equity increased steadily from four in ICME 7 to 8 in ICME 11
- Similarly, the number of groups (working groups, topic groups, discussion groups) pertaining to equity have been increasing steadily since ICME 6 (1988) in Budapest
- In general the results indicate that up to 1988, the focus of the activties of ICME congresses was on quality issues, and since then, the focus on equity increased gradually and steadily

2.3.3 The PME Annual Conferences

The International Group for the Psychology of Mathematics Education (PME) started as a professional organization in 1977 to promote international contacts, exchange, and interdisciplinary research in the psychology of mathematics education. PME has since organized the annual conferences which covered

Lectures		Groups
Plenary	Non-plenary	
ICME1		
None	None	None
ICME 2		
-Mathematical education in developing countries – some problems of teaching and learning (Hugh Philip)	None	-Mathematics in Developing Countries
ICME 3		
-The Interaction between Mathematics and Society (J. Lighthill) - Education in Mathematics and Science Today: The Spread of False Dichotomies (P. Hilton)	None	Not available
ICME 4		
-Experiences in popularizing mathematical methods (Hua Loo-Keng)	None	-Working Group on increasing the participation of women in mathematics
ICME 5		
-Socio-Cultural Bases for Mathematical Education (Ubiratan D'Ambrosio)	None	*Topic Groups* - Women and Mathematics
ICME 6		
-School mathematics in the 1990's: The challenge of change especially for developing countries (Bienvenido Nebres)	None	*Topic Areas* 4: Problems of the handicapped students 13 Women and mathematics *Fifth Day Special: Mathematics, Education, and Society:* -Mathematics education and culture -Society and institutionalized mathematics education -Educational institutions and the individual learner -Mathematics education in the global village

Fig. 2.1. Activities pertaining to equity in ICME congresses 1968–1988

Lectures		Groups
Plenary	Non-plenary	
ICME 7		
None	-A social ethics for math education (Chevallard) - Mathematics education in the global village: the wedge and the filter(Jurdak) - Children and their inherited mathematical culture (Paez) - Mathematics beyond good and evil (Shelley) - New approaches to the mathematical education of minorities in the United States (Treisman)	*Working Groups*: 10: Multicultural and multilingual classrooms 19:Mathematics for pre-mature school leavers 22: Mathematics education with reduced resources *Topic Groups* - Ethnomathematics and math education - Mathematics for work: vocational education - Indigenous peoples and math Education -The social context of math education
ICME 8		
None	- Where does it come from and where does it go? (D'Ambrosio) - Mathematics education and gender issues (Leder)	*Working Groups* 6: Gender and mathematics 7: Mathematics for gifted students 8: Mathematics for special students 21: The teaching of mathematics in different cultures 22: Mathematics, education, society, and culture *Topic Groups* -Education for mathematics in the working place
ICME 9		
None	- Overcoming obstacles to the democratization of math education (Bishop) -The socio-cultural turn in the studying, the teaching, and learning of mathematics (Lerman) - Designing instruction of values in school mathematics (Soedjadi) - Widening the lens- changing the focus: Researching and describing language practices in the multilingual classrooms in South Africa (Adler) - Cultural cross-purposes and expectations as barriers to success in mathematics (Clark) - On the role of politics in the development of mathematics in Africa (El Tom) - In search of an East Asian identity in math education (Leung) - The impact of California? back-to- basics policies (Jacob) - Math education for and in the dominant and the other cultures (Sakonidis)	*Working Groups* -The social and political dimensions of math education -History and culture in math education *Topic Groups* 15: Math education for students with special needs 17: Mathematics education and equity 21:Ethnomathematics

Fig. 2.2. Activities pertaining to equity in ICME congresses 1992–2000

	Lectures		Groups
Plenary		Non-plenary	
		ICME 10	
-Mathematics education for whom and why? The balance between mathematics education for all and for high level mathematics performance (Lerman, Askey, Carreira, Namikawa, Vithal)		-On the relationships between informal out-of-school mathematics and formal in-school mathematics in the development of abstract mathematical knowledge (Bonnotto) -Promoting equity in math education (Baoler) - Globalization, ghettoizing, and uncertainty: Challenges for critical math education (Skovsmose) - Math education and language: policy, research and practice in multilingual contexts (Setati)	*Topic Study Groups* 4: Activities and programmes for gifted students 5: Activities and programmes for students with special needs 6: Adult and life-long mathematics education 7: Math education in and for work *Discussion Groups* 3: Mathematics for whom and why? The balance between 'mathematics education for all' and 'for high level mathematical activity 5: International cooperation in math education 7: Public understanding of mathematics and math education 15 Ethnomathematics Current problems and challenges concerning studets with special needs
		ICME 11	
- Equal access to quality math education (Panel: Bill Atweh (moderator); Olympia Figueras; Murad Jurdak; Catherine Vistr-Yu)		-Challenges to mathematics education research faced by developing countries. Report of Survey Team 2(Borba) -Equity: The Case for and against gender(Leder) -Socio-cultural perspectives on the learning and development of mathematics teachers and teacher-educator-researchers(Goos) -Ethnomathematics at the margin of Europe. A pagan calendar in modern times(Bjarnadóttir) -Mathematics education in multicultural and multilingual environments. Report of Survey Team 5(Bishop) -Mathematical literacy in South Africa – an opportunity for shifting learner identities in relation to mathematics(Graven) -How mathematics education can help in shaping a better world?(D'Ambrosio) -Societal challenges to mathematics education in different countries. Report on Survey Team 6(Ferrini-Mundy)	*Topic Study Group* 6: Activities and programs for gifted students 7: Activities and programs for students with special needs 8: Adult mathematics education 9: Math education in and for work 32: Gender and math education 33: Math education in a multi-linguistic multicultural environments *Discussion Groups* 10: Public perceptions and understanding of mathematics and mathematics education 11: Quality and relevance in mathematics education research 18: The role of ethnomathematics in mathematics education

Fig. 2.3. Activities pertaining to equity in ICME congresses 2004–2008

different aspects of interdisciplinary research in the psychology of mathematics education and other related fields.

In his comprehensive survey and analysis of the evolution of equity and social justice in the PME, Gates (2006) traced these concepts as they appeared in PME proceedings. Based on his survey and analysis, Gates gave the following conclusions:

- In the early years of PME (1977–1986), 'there was a slight attention to issues that relate to the social context in which learners and teachers live and work' (p. 375)
- At the end of the second decade (1987–1996) of PME, more attention was given to equity and social justice as evidenced by the emergence of equity, gender, and ethnomathematics issues in PME research. 'This however has not yet reached the sophistication that theories have reached outside PME research literature-the social systematic level' (p. 84)
- By the third phase of PME (1997–2005), PME research showed a broadened interest in the cultural and social contexts of mathematics learning and teaching such as compatibility between home and school cultures. learning in multilingual context and in indigenous communities.

All in all, PME research seems to have followed the same pattern as ICME's as far as equity in mathematics education is concerned. The 1980s was the decade when interest in social and cultural issues in mathematics education started to emerge. The 1990s was the decade when social and cultural issues became a significant and growing component of research in mathematics education.

2.4 Conclusion

Figure 2.4 presents a summary of the evolution of equity and quality in education and mathematics education in the period 1950–2008. The pattern of evolution of the concepts of equity and quality in mathematics education that emerges from the survey of the literature and ICMI activities differs from the pattern of the evolution of these two concepts that emerges from the survey of the relevant international literature. As to the evolution of the concepts of educational equity and quality, the concept of educational equity in terms of provision for universal primary education was paramount between 1950 and 2000 but educational quality received low priority during that period. In the first decade of the twenty-first century, quality education for all has emerged as a top priority.

On the other hand, the evolution of the concepts of equity and quality in mathematics education was dominated by quality concerns in scholarly discourse between 1950 and 1980. The social and cultural aspects of mathematics education started to emerge as legitimate research in the 1980s. Towards the end of 1980s, equity issues became a major concern in mathematics education.

Period	Education		Math Education	
	Equity	Quality	Equity	Quality
1950's	Universal Primary Education (UPE)	Little emphasis	Little emphasis	Understanding math concepts and processes
1960's	Universal Primary Education (UPE)	Little emphasis	Little emphasis	Understanding math concepts and processes
1970's	Universal Primary Education (UPE)	-Faure's vision of educational quality -Little emphasis in practice	Little emphasis	Questioning the goals of new math
1980's	Universal Primary Education (UPE)	Little emphasis	Little emphasis	Serving adult life, societal, and technological needs
1990's	Universal Primary Education (UPE)	-Delores vision of educational quality -Little emphasis in practice	Math education for all	Quality math education for all
2001–2010	Education for all	Quality education for all	Math education for all	Quality math education for all

Fig. 2.4. Summary of the evolution of equity and quality in education and mathematics education 1950–2008

The first decade of the twenty-first Century witnessed the shift towards an increased emphasis on achieving equal access to quality math education.

3

Equity in Quality: Towards a Theoretical Framework

Chapter 2 dealt with the evolution of equity and quality issues in both education and mathematics education and came to the conclusion that equal access to quality education, which includes mathematics education, has become the focus of research and policy-making. Equity and quality are not only research issues which cut across different disciplines but are conceived as major determinants of socioeconomic and human development in both industrial and developing countries, as evidenced by the annual reports of the United Nations Development Program (UNDP).

The status and role of mathematics, a subject which has long enjoyed a privileged status in school curricula worldwide due to its perceived role in science and technology, render equity and quality in mathematics education crucial to human development. This is reflected by governments' relatively large investments in improving the quality of mathematics education and extending it to marginalized and underprivileged groups.

Mathematics has been described as a filter and a gateway to the professions, science and technology. Research in the last four decades has focused on the identification of inequities in mathematics education, the factors that contribute to them (gender, socioeconomic class, ethnicity, location, special needs), the contexts (school, national, global) that impact equity and social justice, and the ways through which teachers and schools deal with such inequities. The attention given to issues of equity and quality in mathematics education is reflected by recent books and reports on the subject (Atweh, Forgasz, & Nebres, 2001; Burton, 2003; Secada & Byrd-Adajian, 1995; Valero & Zevenbergen, 2004) as well as comparative studies based on international or regional mathematics achievement databases (Hanushek & Luque, 2003; PISA, 2005; Jurdak, 2006).

Numerous calls and proposals have been made and many projects implemented to improve quality in mathematics education. Although such efforts often had a positive impact on the quality of the learning outcomes, these efforts increased or created disparities that led to more inequity in math education. Mathematics educators are concerned about the risk that math

M. Jurdak, *Toward Equity in Quality in Mathematics Education*,
DOI 10.1007/978-1-4419-0558-1_3,
© Springer Science+Business Media, LLC 2009

education quality enhancement may result in different levels of mathematical literacy, and consequently increase the potential of marginalizing certain individuals and groups in the same society.

The growing roles of globalization and Information and Communication Technology (ICT) have increased the tension between equity and quality in mathematics education. The demands of the global economy have increased the gap between developed and developing countries and thus made equity in mathematics education not only a within-country phenomenon but also a global one. On the other hand, the disparities in access to and ownership of ICT, which has become an essential tool for quality improvement in mathematics education, rendered the developing countries at a disadvantage in benefiting equitably from quality improvement in mathematics education.

To demonstrate the different conceptions of equity and quality and the tensions between them, I have selected four quotations from the research literature in mathematics education for the purpose of illustration and discussion.

3.1 Quotations

3.1.1 Quotation 1: Inside and Outside School

This study examines the computational strategies of ten young street vendors in Beirut by describing, comparing, and analyzing the computational strategies used in solving three types of problems in two settings: transactions in the workplace, word problems, and computation exercises in a school-like setting. The results indicate that vendors' use of semantically-based mental computational strategies was more predominant in transactions and word problems than in computation exercises whereas written school-like computational strategies were used more frequently in computation exercises than in word problems and transactions. There was clear evidence of more effective use of logico-mathematical properties in transactions and word problems than in computation exercises. Moreover, the success rate associated with each of transactions and word problems was much higher than that associated with computation exercises. (Jurdak, 1999, p. 155)

Do the street vendors have a better 'quality' in their use of mental computational strategies than school students? Did their disadvantage as far as access to school affect their opportunity to learn mathematics beyond the context of their work?

3.1.2 Quotation 2: In the Same Classroom

In this paper I explore the structuring of English children into learning and life trajectories and the part that mathematics has in this process. Using case reports of two ten-year-olds in their final year of primary school education, I examine how broader family social milieu impacts upon mathematics learning trajectories. Stacey and Edward live not far from one another in a city in the midlands of England and have been in the same class from age 5 to 11 yet their social distance is considerable. Through the mobilization of various classed and classifying responses to school mathematics they have developed two very different perspectives on the value of mathematical study. This examination of mathematical marginalization and unrecognized meritocracy raises questions about the extent to which teachers can disrupt such processes. (Noyes, 2007, p. 35)

Is the quality of mathematics learning affected by factors outside school control (such as family social milieu), even for students who have been in the same school and in the same class for six years? Is the 'social distance' between students a determinant of the quality of mathematics learning regardless of equal opportunities in school?

3.1.3 Quotation 3: Inside and Outside a Country

In this paper, I discuss some links between mathematics education and democracy, what these links could imply to what and how we teach, and the issues that arise from trying to further these links. I first suggest three links between mathematics education and democracy formulated on the basis of experiences in Denmark, in particular: learning to relate to authorities' use of mathematics, learning to act in a democracy, and developing a democratic classroom culture. The first two are discussed in relation to narratives from real life, with a focus on the tensions which they reveal. From the discussion following the first narrative, it is clear that what is a competency in one context may not be so in another. This is supported by the second narrative which also questions what is most relevant to students in South Africa and thereby gives rise to the formulation of a fourth connection between democracy and mathematics education, related to issues of access. The third narrative informs a discussion of what it means to be critical. It also continues to address the potential tension between wanting to promote students' critical skills and a democratic classroom culture versus wanting to support students in learning what others have developed and what is required in order to succeed in the schooling system ... (Christiansen, 2007, p. 49)

Is it that what is valued as significant mathematics learning in one context is perceived as irrelevant and may be offensive in another context? Are the criteria by which we judge the quality of mathematics universal? Consequently, what is the basis for comparing the quality of mathematics learning across countries?

3.1.4 Quotation 4: Across Countries

> With these findings in mind, case studies from eleven countries provide insights into how both rich and developing nations have tackled the quality issue. Four of the eleven – Canada, Cuba, Finland and the Republic of Korea – have achieved high standards of education quality, as measured by international tests. The Republic of Korea is ranked first for science and third for mathematics in PISA, Canada comes second for reading and Finland has the highest overall scores, while in Cuba students' average performance topped countries in the region surveyed in 2002 by OREALC1/UNESCO. (UNESCO, 2005, p. 13)

> Several common strands emerge in the four high performing countries. All hold the teaching profession in high regard and support it with investment in training. There is policy continuity over time and a strong, explicit vision of education's objectives (UNESCO, 2005, p. 14)

How could such four countries, in four different continents and at varying distances from each other economically, socially, culturally, and politically, have achieved 'high standards of education quality'?

The questions that were posed about the quotations do not have easy answers. One might say that these quotations are eclectic summaries of larger papers or that the questions are pointed to suggest certain answers. Despite all of this, the fact is that we do not have reasonable answers to such disturbing questions. However, these questions point to a problem manifested in our lack of sufficiently adequate conceptions of quality and equity and the relationship between them. It is hypothesized that the discrepancies underlined in the previous questions are not likely to be adequately explained by the conceptual model of the school as a production system. In the next section, I describe the school as a production system and demonstrate how these discrepancies relate to the conceptions of equity and quality in that system.

3.2 Equity and Quality in the School as a Production System

3.2.1 The School as a Production System

A well-known conceptual framework for the school is that of a production system (in the industrial sense) where education within the school is viewed as a system embedded in a social context and aims at the transformation of inputs into outputs through school processes. Figure 3.1 represents the model of the school as a production system (PISA, 2005). Some examples of the elements of the school as a production system are given below:

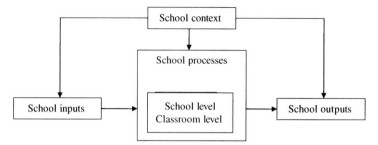

Fig. 3.1. Model of how schools function

School inputs: Learner characteristics, entry aptitudes and skills of teachers and staff, material resources.

School processes: Organization, administration, governance, leadership, climate.

Classroom processes: Teaching, learning and assessment

School context: School socioeconomic-cultural context, educational system context, political system context

School outputs: Literacy, numeracy, life skills, creative skills, values, social benefits

The role of school context in the production system is ideally supposed to be a source of both inputs and constraints. It is often the case that the school context is viewed as a source of constraints rather than inputs. This gave rise to the 'deficit model', which assumes that the incompatibility between the student socioeconomic and cultural contexts, and school demands is a deficit to be compensated for by the school.

Mathematics education is a subsystem of the school system. Consequently, in mathematics education as a production system, the elements of inputs, context, and school processes would be those of the school production system as a whole; however, classroom processes and outputs are mathematics-specific: classroom processes would be the teaching, learning, and assessment of mathematics and the outputs would be the learning outcomes in mathematics.

3.2.2 Equity in the Production System

Educational equity is a fundamental concept which has its basis in ideology, sociology, epistemology, and psychology. It is not surprising therefore that educational equity has assumed different meanings over the years (Sriraman, 2007). Both the concept 'equity' and its label have been challenged lately by many researchers who proposed 'social justice' as an alternative on philosophical and ideological grounds (Burton, 2003).

Berne and Stiefel (1984) proposed a framework for equity in school systems. The framework consists of three components:

1. *Targets of equity concerns*: Gender, socioeconomic status, ethnicity, disability status...
2. *Objects of equity*: Access, resources, and outputs
3. *Principles of equity*: Principles to analyze equity across individuals, regions, countries...

Berne and Stiefel (1984) provided three different principles of equity:

Horizontal equity: Horizontal equity requires that students who are equally situated be equally treated by ensuring that they experience similar levels of human and material resources and hopefully achieve similar outcomes.

Vertical equity: Vertical equity requires differentiation of provision of resources according to individual characteristics in the sense that students who are differently situated would be provided with unique resources (e.g. support programs) to achieve similar results.

Equal opportunity: Equal Educational Opportunity (EEQ) is based on the notion that all students should be given equal chances to succeed. This requires that students should have access to resources that equalizes their starting point and to provide the conditions that allow the possibility of success for all.

This framework seems to be applicable to mathematics education as a production system; however, the equity targets and equity objects are defined to suit mathematics education. The equity targets in education (gender, socioeconomic status, ethnicity, disability status...) apply to mathematics education. In addition, mathematics education may have other mathematics-specific targets such as language of instruction and the use of ICT in mathematics learning.

3.2.3 Quality in the Production System

There are different definitions of quality in education on different philosophical, psychological, social, and discipline-specific perspectives. Quality is closely related to our conceptions of learning. Sfard (1998) proposed that learning theories fall under two learning metaphors, acquisition and participation. In the acquisition metaphor, the individual mind is viewed as a container and thus learning is a matter of acquisition of knowledge. In the participation model, learning is viewed as a process of participation in cultural practices and shared activities, and the emphasis is on the process of knowing and on participating in it, rather than on products such as knowledge and outcomes. In mathematics education, the two metaphors are reflected in mathematics-specific perspectives of quality.

Acquisition Metaphor

Discipline-based perspective: Mathematics education is of good quality in as much as it reflects truthfully the concepts, principles, structure, and mode of thinking of mathematics.

System perspective: Mathematics education is of good quality in as much as the components of the system of mathematics education i.e. inputs, processes and outputs are judged to have good quality.

Participation Metaphor

Meaning-construction perspective: Mathematics education is of good quality in as much as it allows students to individually (or socially) construct the meaning of mathematical concepts and principles.

Critical Theory perspective: Mathematics education is of good quality in as much as it encourages the use of mathematics for the purpose of the critical analysis of social power relationships and production and transmission of formal knowledge.

Indigenous perspective: Mathematics education is of good quality in as much as it enables the individual to build his/her own knowledge, based on indigenous accessible informal knowledge in the learner's social-cultural context e.g. ethnomathematics

The quality of the output is at the core of the quality of the school as a production system. Six variations of quality in the production system are often cited (PISA, 2005). The first is the *productivity* view, which translates in the case of mathematics education to saying that the quality of mathematics education depends on the degree of the attainment of the desired outcomes. The second is the *instrumental* view which assumes that the quality of mathematics education is contingent on the optimal selection of inputs, processes, and contexts that increase the chances of improving performance on outcomes. The third perspective is the *efficiency* view which defines quality in terms of achieving the highest output at the lowest possible cost. The fourth perspective is the *adaptive* view which stipulates that the quality of mathematics education is inherent in its ability to change as a result of critical analysis of its goals of teaching. The fifth perspective is the *equity* view which makes the equal or fair distribution of inputs, processes and outcomes a prerequisite for the quality of mathematics education. The last perspective is the *disjointed* view. This view assumes that the quality of mathematics education depends on the performance of specified aspects of mathematics education, such as teacher training or teaching strategies.

3.2.4 Revisiting the Quotations from the Perspective of the Production System

The discrepancies in the conceptions of equity and quality in the four quotations do not seem to be satisfactorily explained by the school as a production system. Quotation 1 illustrates that the production system does not adequately explain the superior performance in computational strategies of young street vendors, compared to that of students since it does not recognize learning mathematics in an out-of-school social context.

In Quotation 2, seemingly, Stacey and Edward had equal opportunities to learn mathematics. However, they have different valuation of their mathematics learning because of the difference in their cultural capital due to differences in family social milieu. Thus the seemingly equitable inputs and processes in the school did not result in comparable quality of their mathematics learning trajectories. Thus, even in the same school, differences in quality, due to social factors, can not be accounted for by the school as a production system.

Quotation 3 illustrates the difference in conception of quality in two different cultures. What is valued as a mathematics goal in Denmark (learning to relate to authorities' use of mathematics, learning to act in a democracy, and developing a democratic classroom culture) is not considered valuable in South Africa which has a hard-earned democratic political system. This difference in the democracy-related goals of mathematics education reflects different conceptions of quality attributed to ideological factors not accounted for by the school production system framework.

Quotation 4 illustrates that quality, even if it is narrowly defined as the performance on an achievement test, is not necessarily dependent on material resources of the country but rather on its cultural values such as holding the teaching profession in high regard and supporting it with investment in training and the political system and its vision such as policy continuity over time and a strong, explicit vision of the objectives of education.

3.2.5 Comments on Equity and Quality in the School as a Production System

The issue with the production system is that it does not capture the complexity of the social, cultural, and political contexts of mathematics education. First, the school context in the production system has a one-way contribution to the system (Figure 3.1) and does not encompass the broader social-cultural context. Second, the system is not cognizant of the community of learners and the cultural capital they bring to the learning process. Third, placing so much emphasis on the quality of the outcomes is likely to make it a closed system with limited responsiveness to change and innovation because its ultimate aim is improving its productivity and efficiency. Fourth, the ability of the system to manipulate inputs and processes appears to make it responsive to equity concerns. However, this responsiveness remains constrained to surface and macro level indicators such as access, resources, and processes and does not extend to social and cultural equity concerns of individual students.

I suggest that the former apparent discrepancies in conceptions of quality and equity and the relationship between them emanate from two sources. First, equity and quality in mathematics education are aspects of a complex social-cultural-political activity, and second, the theoretical framework of the school as a production system does not capture the nature of mathematics education as a social-cultural-political activity. We suggest a theoretical framework that may address the aforementioned shortcomings of the production system. This framework is based on activity theory as developed by Leont'ev (1981) and activity system as developed by Engeström (1987).

3.3 Activity Theory and Mathematics Education

Because the production model does not seem to capture the nature of mathematics education as a social-cultural-political activity, we propose the activity system as an alternative model. We first introduce activity theory (Leont'ev, 1981) on the basis of which the construct of activity system (Engeström, 1987) was built. Then we demonstrate how we can look at mathematics education as an activity system.

3.3.1 Activity Theory

Activity theory was developed by Leont'ev (1981). He defines activity as:

> ...the unit of life that is mediated by mental reflection. The real function of this unit is to orient the subjects in the world of objects. In other words, activity is not a reaction or aggregate of reactions, but a system with its own structure, its own internal transformations, and its own development. (p. 46)

A central assertion of activity theory is that our knowledge of the world is mediated by our interaction with it, and thus, human behavior and thinking occur within meaningful contexts as people conduct purposeful goal-directed activities. This theory strongly advocates socially organized human activity as the major unit of analysis in psychological studies rather than mind or behavior.

Leont'ev (1981) identified several interrelated levels or abstractions in activity theory. Each level is associated with a special type of unit. The first most general level is associated with the unit of activity that deals with specific real activities such as work, play, and learning. The second level of analysis focuses on the unit of a goal-directed action that is the process subordinated to a conscious goal. The third level of analysis is associated with the unit of operation or the conditions under which the action is carried out. Operations help actualize the general goal to make it more concrete.

Human activity can be realized in two forms: Mental or internal activity and practical objective or external activity (Leont'ev, 1981). The fundamental and primary form of human activity is external and practical. This form of activity brings humans into practical contact with objects thus redirecting, changing and enriching this activity. The internal plane of activity is formed as a result of internalizing external processes.

"Internalization is the transition in which external processes with external, material objects are transformed into processes that take place at the mental level, the level of consciousness" (Zinchencho & Gordon, 1981, p. 74)

Three types of actions in mental activities had been identified: Perceptual, mnemonic, and cognitive (Zinchencho & Gordon, 1981). Perceptual actions are those through which the human being maintains contact with the environment. They are initiated by stimuli from the environment and enriched on the basis of prior experience. Mnemonic actions refer to actions that involve recognition, reconstruction, or recall (Piaget & Inhelder as cited in Zinchencho & Gordon, 1981). Cognitive actions involve thinking in terms of images of real objective processes (Gal'perin cited in Zinchencho & Gordon, 1981).

3.3.2 Activity System

Engeström (1987) developed the construct of activity system to describe and account for the collective (as compared to individual) human activity in the broad historical-cultural-social contexts. Figure 3.2 is a schematic diagram of the activity structure as developed by Engeström (1999). The activity system has the following elements:

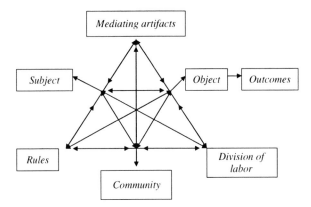

Fig. 3.2. The structure of human activity

Object: The object is the problem space targeted by the activity of the organization and this goal-object is transformed into outcomes.
Subject: The subject refers to an individual (individual activity) or a group (collective activity) in an organization.
Mediating artifacts: The mediating artifacts are cultural products that act as intermediary or auxiliary in effecting the appropriation of the cultural aspects embodied in these products. The mediating artifacts consist of

physical and symbolic, external and internal mediating instruments, including both tools and signs.

Community: The community represents those individuals and or subgroups
that share the same general object of the activity and define themselves
as distinct from other communities.

Rules: The rules are the explicit and implicit regulations, norms, and conventions that regulate and control the actions and the interactions within the
activity.

Division of labor: The division of labor refers to both the division of tasks
between members of the community and to the division of power and
authority within the activity.

3.3.3 Mathematics Education as an Activity System

Figure 3.3 is a schematic diagram of mathematics education as an activity
in the classroom at the level of the school system. In the next paragraph
we illustrate how the activity system may be used to describe mathematics
education in the the classroom.

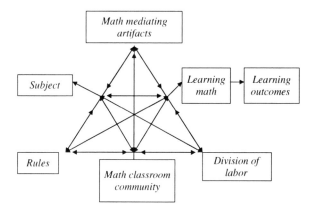

Fig. 3.3. The structure of mathematics education activity

In the classroom, the object of mathematics education as an activity system is the learning of mathematics. The learning of mathematics is transformed into learning outcomes by the help of the mediating artifacts which
are used in the classroom and include mathematical and non-mathematical
physical tools such as the computer or symbolic tools like language and mathematical symbols. The community which consists of those individuals which
share the same object of learning mathematics includes the students in the
class as well as the teacher. The division of labor refers to division of tasks as
well as division of authority among the students and teachers while trying to
achieve the object of the activity. The rules consist of explicit school regulations as well as implicit school and wider-scale social norms and conventions.

3.3.4 Mathematics Education as a Nested Hierarchical Complex Activity System

The activity system of mathematics education is a complex nested hierarchical 3-layer system: The school activity system, the national activity system, and the global system (Figure 3.4). Each system is nested within the next higher one: The school system plays the role of the 'subject' in the national system and similarly the national system plays the role of the 'subject' in the global system. One implication of this nested hierarchical structure is that the societal relationships of power and influence of a higher system carry over to the lower systems and eventually to the student activity system at the classroom level. What is common to the activity sub-systems in the three nested contexts (school, nation, world) is that they share a common object i.e learning of mathematics, but not necessarily the same mathematics learning outcomes.

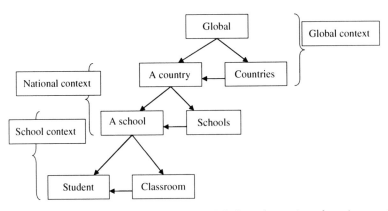

Fig. 3.4. Structure of school, country, and global mathematics education contexts

From another perspective, mathematics education may be viewed as an activity system that exists concurrently with other systems sharing the same context but having different objects. For example, in the same classroom, the mathematics education subsystem exists concurrently with a science activity subsystem that has the same community but a different object (learning of science).

3.4 Equity and Quality in the Activity System

In this section, we present the conceptions of equity, quality, and the relationship between them from the perspective of the activity system framework.

3.4.1 Equity in the Activity System

In the production model the equity concerns were viewed as single factors such as gender, socioeconomic status, ethnicity, disability status. The activity system factors are by themselves neutral to equity or inequity; *it is the interaction of these factors with other factors* that may render them inequitable. For example, at the classroom level, the factor of gender (a factor which belongs to the student) is neutral as far as equity is concerned. However, if and when the two genders are treated differently in terms of use of computers (a factor which belongs to mathematics mediating artifacts) gender becomes a factor which affects equity among students in mathematics learning in the classroom. At the country level, the constituency of a school is not an inequity factor between schools. However, if schools with different constituencies have different levels of achievement, the school constituency becomes an inequity factor.

The factors of the activity system are related horizontally and longitudinally. Horizontally, for each level of the activity system (school, national, and global), inequities are due to the interactions among the other factors in the system. Longitudinally, the elements of a system at one level are related to the elements of the system at another level by a hierarchical relation of inclusion. For example, gender is a factor under 'student' in the school system and as such it interacts with other factors in the mathematics education activity system at the school level to produce inequities. On the other hand, if gender as an inequity factor becomes prevalent in many schools, it may become an inequity factor among schools in the mathematics education system at the country level.

The definition of inequity factor as an interaction among activity system factors implies that inequity factors are amenable to change by changing the policies or practices related to that factor. In other words, inequities are generated by interactions among factors and can be reduced also by actions on the same factors. For example, the so-called gender achievement gap in mathematics is viewed as a result of interactions among different factors such as differential treatment between genders in using computers (mediating artifacts) or in classroom participation. This inequity may be addressed by changing the policies or practices regarding computer use and classroom participation.

3.4.2 Quality in the Activity System

Quality in the production system refer to the quality of its outputs or less often to the quality of its inputs, processes, or even the context in which production occurs. Quality in the activity system is closely related to the knowledge creation metaphor of learning which differs from the two metaphors of the acquisition and the participation (Paavola, Lipponen, & Hakkarainen, 2004). According to Paavola et al., the ultimate aim of the knowledge creation models (including Engeström's activity system) is the development of innovative knowledge communities through learning:

"Learning is not conceptualized through processes occurring in individuals' minds, or through processes of participation in social practices. Learning is understood as a collaborative effort directed toward developing some mediated artifacts, broadly defined as including knowledge, ideas, practices, and material or conceptual artifacts. The interaction among different forms of knowledge or between knowledge and other activities is emphasized as a requirement for this kind of innovative learning and knowledge creation." (p. 569)

In relation to the activity system, Engeström (1999) introduced the model of *expansive cycle* in work teams. The expansive cycle is a qualitative *transformation of the activity system as a whole*. The expansive cycle starts from some *dialectical tension* between the different nodes in the activity system. The change starts at the level of the *individual* members of the community, through the processes of *internalization* and *externalization*. The successful orchestration of the collective emerging individual activities will be an expansive cycle which eventually transforms the system into one which is free of the tension that started it. The transformed system has now different relations and interactions among its components. Here is an example of expansive learning in the school context. In a school, the administration and teachers were *dissatisfied* with the intensity of competition in math among students. The school decides to introduce cooperative learning as a way to develop a spirit of cooperation among students. A cooperative learning professional development program is implemented in the school (this is the start of *internalization*). Following the training, the teachers start to implement cooperative learning in their math classroom teaching. As they do so, each *individual* teacher engages in a process to optimize cooperative learning to the actual conditions of the classroom (this is the start of *externalization*). The teachers may have different ways of meeting the specific needs of their students. As they progress in externalizing their learning based on their experience, they come closer to *appropriating* cooperative learning in the routines of their teaching. The school administration monitors the individual teachers' optimization efforts and tries to synthesize them into one coherent policy. If the policy is adapted and practiced by all school teachers, then that school system has achieved an expansive cycle, i.e has been qualitatively transformed.

3.4.3 The Activity System and the Social-Cultural-Political Nature of Math Education

The criterion of quality of mathematics education from the perspective of the activity system does not reside in the quality of its output (learning outcomes) or in the quality of the inputs or the processes of the system. Quality in the activity system is the extent of the responsiveness to which the system as a whole responds and adapts to emerging needs, thus transforming itself and expanding into a new one.

The dialectical relationship between equity and equality in the activity system seems to capture the social-cultural-political nature of mathematics education. From the perspective of the activity system, the inequities that appear in the system because of social, cultural, or political reasons act as de-stabilizing factors. According to expansive learning, the tension thus produced will make the system more responsive to social-cultural-political concerns of mathematics education. This responsiveness takes the form of re-structuring the system to address these inequities.

3.4.4 Revisiting the Quotations from the Perspective of Activity System

In this section we reexamine the quotations from the perspective of the activity system to find out whether this system, compared to the production system, contributes to a better understanding of the discrepancies we identified earlier. In Quotation 1, the discrepancies regarding equity and quality between street vendors and students may be accounted for, from the perspective of activity theory, by the observation that equity and quality are not comparable in the two cases since the street vendors and students are operating in two different activity systems. In the case of vendors, the workplace activity system con-sists of subjects (vendors) who are working in a community of other vendors and customers whose object is selling or buying produce, using all mediated artifacts (calculations and other physical tools), utilizing agreed upon division of labor, and operating within the rules of the local market and the acceptable social norms and conventions. On the other hand, the school activity system consists of a community of students and teachers whose object in the mathe-matics classroom is the learning of mathematics, using mediated artifacts and division of labor determined and limited by the school, and operating within the rules and policies of the school and social conventions of the larger school community.

In Quotation 2, the fact that equal opportunities to learn mathematics afforded to Stacey and Edward did not lead to a comparable valuation of their mathematics learning may be accounted for by the interaction of social-cultural capital (rules) and the relation of each of Stacey and Edward to the object of learning mathematics.

In Quotation 3, the difference in the conception of quality in the two cul-tures of Denmark and South Africa may also be explained by the activity sys-tem framework. What is valued as a desirable object for learning mathematics in Denmark (learning to relate to authorities' use of mathematics, learning to act in a democracy, and developing a democratic classroom culture) is not con-sidered a valuable outcome of the activity of learning mathematics in South Africa. This discrepancy may be accounted for in terms of the interaction of the 'community' and 'object' components of the activity system.

In Quotation 4, the four countries - Canada, Cuba, Finland and the Re-public of Korea - have achieved, according to UNESCO, high standards of educational quality, which was attributed to the fact that these countries shared some cultural similarities (holding the teaching profession in high regard and supporting it with investment in training) as well as political similarities (policy continuity over time and a strong, explicit vision of education's objectives). Both the cultural and political aspects shared by the four countries belong to the 'rules' in the activity system.

In this book, the activity system will be used as a theoretical framework to identify and analyze the factors that contribute to equity and quality in mathematics education. In the next three chapters, the activity systems of math education at the school, country, and global levels will be introduced and exemplified. Moreover, these three chapters will review and analyze relevant literature on equity in math education at the school, country, and global levels, using the lens of the activity system.

In Part II of the book, the TIMSS assessment and the background questionnaires data will be used to identify student, teacher, school, and country contextual variables which impact math achievement. The activity system will be used to interpret the identified contextual variables as inequity factors.

4

The School Context

This chapter focuses on identifying and analyzing the factors in the school context that may generate inequities in mathematics education. The chapter is organized as follows. First, it describes the activity system associated with mathematics education at this level and identifies the factors (nodes of the activity system) and their attributes, that may contribute to inequities in mathematics education at this level. Second, it reviews and synthesizes the equity-related mathematics education research from journals, conference proceedings, and books, in an attempt to draw a profile of the research findings regarding the inequities that result from the interactions of the attributes of the activity system factors.

4.1 Math Education System at the School Level: Factors and Their Attributes

Figure 4.1, identifies the factors that belong to each of the six nodes of the activity system which are likely to interact to produce inequities. There are two kinds of inequity factors, those that *directly* impact math learning and those that impact it indirectly. For example the inequity factors that result from the interaction of student attributes and mediating artifacts attributes impact mathematics learning directly, whereas the inequity factors that result from the interaction of student attributes and rules impact learning of mathematics indirectly.

What follows is a brief description, with examples, of each factor and its relevant attributes as they relate to the activity system of mathematics education at the school level. The titles of the six subsections correspond to to the six factors (nodes) as they appear in Figure 4.1.

M. Jurdak, *Toward Equity in Quality in Mathematics Education*,
DOI 10.1007/978-1-4419-0558-1_4,
© Springer Science+Business Media, LLC 2009

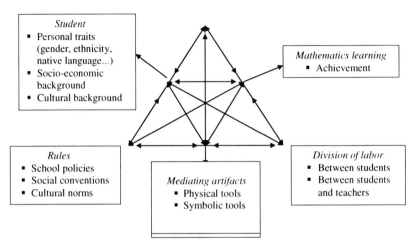

Fig. 4.1. Factors and their attributes in the activity system of mathematics education at the school level

4.1.1 Mathematics Learning

Since the object of the activity system at the school level is the learning of mathematics, the whole system is geared towards that. The object of mathematics learning is translated into concrete outcomes such as skills, abilities, concepts, and attitudes. These outcomes are far from being universal, but the learning of mathematics, irrespective of the meaning associated with it, is the universal object of the activity of math education at the school level. The extent to which math learning outcomes are achieved defines how successful the system is in realizing its object.

4.1.2 Student

The individual student in a classroom assumes the role of the 'subject' in the activity system. Research findings have indicated that certain attributes of the student are related to inequities in mathematics learning in the classroom. The student's personal traits are those characteristics the student is born with, such as the student's ethnic group, gender, and native language. Although the student's personal traits are not amenable to change, the meaning one attributes to them is socially constituted.

The student's socioeconomic background is an attribute that may impact mathematics learning and hence affect equity in the opportunity of learning and succeeding in math. Many factors contribute to the student's socioeconomic background, such as the income of the student's family compared to the average national income, the occupation of the parents and their educational level, among other things.

A third attribute that may impact equity in mathematics education is the student's cultural background. Many factors contribute to the student's cultural background, such as the value system at home and in the community, the traditions and social norms, the home use of cultural artifacts, especially language and technology.

4.1.3 Classroom Community

The classroom community consists of fellow students and the teacher, all of whom are trying to realize the object of the activity on an ongoing basis. One basic attribute of the classroom community is the constituency of this community in terms of students' socioeconomic and cultural backgrounds. The constituency of the classroom community is one determinant of the social and cultural norms in the classroom.

The organization of the classroom community refers to the different modalities of organizing students' learning of mathematics in the classroom. Among other things, the organization of the classroom community includes different ways of student grouping for learning, codes of behavior, and power relations in the classroom.

The types of acceptable interactions among the classroom community may have a differential impact on mathematics learning and hence on equity in math education. Classroom interactions include teacher-student, student-student, and teacher-class interactions.

4.1.4 Mediating Artifacts

As stated earlier, the mediating artifacts are cultural products that have accumulated as a result of the evolution of a specific culture. These artifacts are symbolic and physical tools which act as intermediary agents in effecting the internalization of the meanings they carry and the externalization of their use in new contexts. Perhaps the most important symbolic artifact is language. Many issues in mathematics learning are related to the language of instruction of mathematics, such as teaching math in a foreign language or having multilingual classrooms. The language of mathematics is another symbolic artifact that may impact mathematics learning. Concrete learning materials, textbooks, and computers are physical artifacts that mediate math teaching and learning.

4.1.5 Division of Labor

This division refers to the way both labor and power are divided through mutual agreement among the members of the classroom community. This division of labor is a tacit understanding by the community members. It is a necessary condition for engaging in the activity and realizing its object because the learning of math in the classroom is a collective activity, and thus each member is expected to have a role in realizing the object of this activity. In the classroom, the division of labor takes place among the students themselves, the teacher and the students, or student groups and the teacher.

4.1.6 Rules

The function of rules is that they govern the interactions between the student and the school community, and as such impact indirectly other interactions in the system. The rules are of two types. One type relates to the explicit rules set by the school in the form of policies and regulations and the other relates to more ubiquitous rules that emanate from the social conventions and cultural norms.

4.2 Interactions and Inequities: Two Examples

Inequities in mathematics education at the school level are potentially generated by the interactions of the attributes of the factors in the activity system. Figure 4.1 identifies the salient factors that belong to the six nodes of the activity system. These factors by themselves are neutral to equity or inequity; it is the interaction of these factors that may render them inequitable. The interactions of such factors or their attributes will be called *inequity factors*.

An example of how attributes or factors interact to generate inequities in the activity system at the school level is provided by Noyes (2007). The author illustrates how the social and cultural backgrounds (belong to the 'student' in the activity system) of two English students who lived in the same neighborhood and who had been attending the same class in the same school for six years produced inequities in their valuation of mathematics in school and life (belongs to 'mathematics learning' in the activity system) (see Chapter 3 for more details on this article).

A hypothetical example is presented to illustrate the interaction between student attributes and the math mediating artifacts. Consider two students who go to the same school. One student comes from a working class family and the other from a middle class family. The working class family does not own a computer at home, whereas the middle class family does. The school happens to use computers in teaching mathematics. Obviously, the middle class student has an advantage in using computers over the working class student. This advantage may lead to an advantage in learning mathematics since research has indicated that computer use would have a positive effect on mathematics achievement if it is used at both home and school (see Chapter 8). Consequently, it is likely that the difference in the socioeconomic backgrounds of the two students would result in differential computer use, which, in turn, may affect the level of mathematics achievement.

The rest of the chapter is organized into sections under the following titles:

1. Inequities Related to Student, Mediating Artifacts, and Division of Labor Interactions
2. Inequities Related to Student, Classroom, and Mathematics Achievement Interactions
3. Inequities Related to School Policies and Sociocultural Context

4.3 Inequities Related to Student, Mediating Artifacts, and Division of Labor Interactions

In this section, the interactions between attributes of the 'student' and 'mediating artifacts' will be presented in three sub-sections under which the research issues addressed in the literature will be identified and described.

4.3.1 Student Personal Traits and Mathematics Mediating Artifacts in the Classroom

The literature has addressed, to varying degrees, the inequity factors related to student personal traits (gender, ethnicity, color) and physical mediating artifacts. The inequity factor of gender in relation to IT was addressed only recently with the emergence of computers as powerful teaching and learning resources in mathematics education. Gender-related differences in student beliefs about the efficacy of computers in mathematics learning were addressed by Forgasz (2003) and Vale, Leder, and Forgasz (2003) and to Forgasz (2004). Teachers' attitudes towards the use of computers in secondary mathematics classes reflected gender-related differences in their beliefs regarding their confidence and ability in using computers in mathematics classes (Forgasz, 2006). Ethnicity and native language are closely related and the latter may be considered a personal trait. One strand of research has focused on the learning of mathematics in multilingual classrooms, where the language of instruction is not the native language of the majority. Khisty and Chval (1990) investigated children's language and the communication of mathematical ideas in Hispanic classrooms in the USA. Setati and Adler (2001) studied language practices in multilingual mathematics classrooms in South Africa. Towards the end of the last century, language research shifted towards studying the potential exclusionary role of multicultural, multilingual societies (Barwell, 2001; Setati, 2003) including classrooms with a high percentage of immigrants (Gorgorio & Planas, 2001). Others tried to develop theoretical frameworks for the role of cultural, language and discursive practices in the mathematics classroom (Lerman, 2003). Moreover, multiple language use in mathematics classrooms has been increasingly interpreted from a political perspective (Gustein, 2007).

The mathematics textbook is another artifact which may generate gender-related inequities. For example, the language and contexts in mathematics textbooks may favor one gender over the other or even ignore one gender altogether in countries where co-education is not practiced. Needless to say, the inequities are compounded when the language of the textbook is not the native language. In general, research has rarely addressed gender-related differences in mathematics textbooks.

In summary the dominant inequity factors due to the interaction of student factors and mediating artifacts seem to be dominated by two factors. One is the result of interaction of student gender and the use of technology and the second results from the interaction of the student's native language and multilingual mathematics classrooms.

4.3.2 Student Socioeconomic Background and Mathematics Mediating Artifacts in the Classroom

Social theories differ in their justification of the well-documented conclusion that the student socioeconomic background is a critical inequity factor in mathematics education. Some social theories hypothesize that inequities in education associated with social class can be explained by the inequitable distribution of resources in schools and classrooms. Other critical social theories attribute social class inequities in education to deeper social power and culture. Bourdieu, Passeron, and de saint Martin (1994) introduced the concept of habitus which is the concrete embodiment of culture in the form of thoughts, actions, and behaviors. Many studies have hypothesized that social class differences are often associated with differences in familial and home habitus. Researchers, including Bourdieu, hypothesize that in countries where distinct class differences exist, the school classroom habitus reflects the home habitus of the more powerful social classes. The dissonance between the classroom habitus and the home habitus of the low socioeconomic class is normally the largest because that class has the least power. Consequently, pedagogic practices favor students from dominant upper social classes over students coming from a low socioeconomic background, in terms of participation, engagement, and meaningful learning of mathematics. In a sense the low socioeconomic class students may be regarded metaphorically as 'immigrants' in the mathematics classroom and, as such, experience the same difficulties that immigrants face in foreign countries, especially in their use of the mathematics mediating artifacts that constitute the classroom habitus. From the perspective of critical social theories, the student's social class is a potent inequity factor in relation to the symbolic mediating artifacts used in mathematics, especially the language of instruction. Students coming from low social class families are at a disadvantage in negotiating mathematical meaning during classroom discourse and in effective participation in learning mathematics. Zevenbergen (2001) argues that the low socioeconomic class students are disadvantaged, in comparison with middle class students, in that the home linguistic habitus of the latter is more congruous with the mathematics classroom linguistic habitus and predisposes the middle class students to act in line with what is valued by the system.

Social class may also act as an inequity factor in using physical mathematics mediating artifacts. The mathematics textbook may act as an inequity factor in its language as well in the problem solving contexts used in it. The math textbook may disfavor a particular class, often the working class, over other upper classes by including problem situations that are more familiar, and hence more meaningful to students from one social class than to those in the other. Needless to say, the inequities are compounded when the language of the textbook is not the native language.

The availability and appropriation of resources for mathematics instruction and learning are also factors that impact the use of these mediating artifacts in learning and obviously disadvantage low socioeconomic students. Adler (2001), concludes from a study conducted in South Africa that the availability and even the use of resources traditionally used in mathematics classrooms (textbooks and chalkboards) are no guarantee that teachers appropriate these resources by adapting to the needs of their work contexts. According to Adler (2001)

> "... *in contexts of greatest need* [*italics is in the original*] the effects of teachers' appropriation from their in-service experiences and of the recontextualization of new or existing resources perhaps exacerbated inequality." p. 107

Social class acts as an inequity factor in the ownership and appropriation of computers. It is well-known that students of low socioeconomic level are disadvantaged as far as the ownership and appropriation of computers at home. Research has indicated that the use of computers at *both* school and home has a more positive impact on students' mathematics achievement than using them at school only (see Chapter 8 in this book). Hence the use of computers for mathematics instruction in schools is likely to disadvantage low socioeconomic students who normally have little opportunities to own and use computers at home.

In summary the inequity factor of social class in relation to physical and symbolic mathematics mediating artifacts is a powerful one. The availability of the material artifacts is partially under the control of schools. However, the appropriation of symbolic artifacts is not amenable to change by school or even state policies. Language practices in particular are deeply rooted in the social structure of the broader school community.

4.3.3 Student Cultural Background and Mathematics Mediating Artifacts in the Classroom

The factor of culture in relation to mathematics classroom mediating artifacts has been recently recognized as a legitimate and powerful aspect of inequity. Cultural values and practices that are embedded in the broader school community may interact with the mediating artifacts to facilitate or impede learning of math. After all, the mediating artifacts are cultural products and their compatibility with the local culture is an important factor in learning math.

Where and how does the student's cultural background come into the picture as an inequity factor? Obviously the answer to this question relates to the use of cultural products in the classroom. One extreme form of culture-related inequity in mathematics education is 'cultural deprivation', represented by the the de-contextualization of mathematics education, thus depriving students of the opportunity to give meaning to their mathematical learning. An example of cultural deprivation is the formal and rote teaching of counting in elementary school without capitalizing on counting practices used in local communities. Another form of culture-related inequities in mathematics education is 'cultural hegemony', reflected in the over-representation of the practices and artifacts of a specific culture. One example of cultural hegemony is teaching math in a foreign language. Between these two extremes there are many forms of culture-related inequities in mathematics education.

The school's broader sociocultural context consists of at least two interrelated components: The home culture or habitus (Bourdieu et al., 1994) which consists of the thoughts, actions and behaviors practiced at home, and the culture at large, which includes ideological, sociological, sentimental, and technological artifacts and practices (White, 1959). There are two diverging perspectives as to the role of the sociocultural load that the student brings to the mathematics classroom. The critical perspective, represented by Bourdieu, views this cultural load as 'capital' that empowers the student. The failure to invest this capital in learning is the fault of classroom teaching or school processes because the school culture reflects the culture of the dominant social class. On the other hand, the deficit model perspective looks at this cultural load as 'baggage' which may constrain learning and hence is looked at as a shortcoming that should be remedied.

The cultural 'load' carried over by the student to the mathematics classroom and likely to impact equity in mathematics education includes values, cultural practices, and artifacts. Values are the lenses through which students view reality, including mathematics and its teaching. Inequities in the mathematics classroom may arise from perceptions of conflict between mathematical practices and ideological values (Jurdak, 1989), insensitivity towards the values of others, or the inability of teachers to capitalize on shared values in the multi-cultural classroom. Research on values in mathematics education has focused on the identification of relevant student and teacher values, differences in teacher values, and how these differences are reflected in classroom practices and how to optimize instruction to accommodate value differences (Seah, 2004).

Any discussion of cultural artifacts is incomplete without reference to *ethnomathematics*. According to Stillman and Bilatti (2001), ethnomathematics has evolved from its initial formulation by D'Ambrosio (1985) as the study of implicit mathematics within cultural practices in traditional societies (Gerdes, 1988), to a study which elaborates the cultural, social, and political dimensions among identifiable cultural groups in any society, including modern industrial communities (Vithal & Skovsmose, 1997).

The tension between mathematical practices of students in the academic context of the classroom and that outside school may be a source of inequity. The literature lends support to the hypothesis that working class students are quite capable of engaging in higher order mathematical processes in meaningful activities outside the school, whereas they are not able to cope with the 'academic' mathematics in the school (Povey & Boylan, 1998). In a study investigating the lack of engagement of many students in middle school mathematics classes, Sullivan, Tobias, and Mcdonough (2006) report that classroom culture may be an important determinant of under-participation in mathematics classrooms. There is also evidence that the classroom culture does not promote meaningful learning and application of mathematics as much as the culture of the workplace or the real world contexts do (Pozzi, Noss, & Hoyles, 1998; Jurdak & Shahin, 1999; Baker & Street, 2000). Cobb and Hodge (2002) presented a relational perspective on cultural diversity and equity. They analyzed, compared, and contrasted the practices of students' local home communities, the broader communities to which they belonged, and the mathematical practices in the classroom. The authors concluded that students' access to educational and economic opportunities is not limited to their knowledge and participation in out-of-school practices, but is also affected by students' attempts to reconcile their self-concept and aspirations with the identities they are invited to construct in the mathematics classroom. Some mathematics educators attempted interventions which incorporate culturally relevant teaching. For example, Mathews (2003) identified the difficulties in incorporating culturally relevant mathematics teaching in black schools in Bermuda.

Some authors have brought forward the argument that the definitions of equity, access, and student participation in mathematics learning have to be reconsidered as a result of the impact of computers and communication on learning (Wilburg, 2003). It is clear by now that ICT has permeated home and work environments and impacted cultural mathematical practices in such environments. These changes in the out-of-school culture are bound to be reflected in the classroom culture. There is little research on these emerging issues.

In summary, although the students' cultural background has not received attention in research until recently, it has proved to be a powerful inequity factor as far as mathematics mediating artifacts are concerned. It seems that the cultural background of the student acts as an inequity factor if students of different cultures are deprived of the opportunity of seeking mathematical meaning in culturally-relevant situations or if the cultural practices and artifacts of one group are over-represented at the expense of those of other groups.

4.3.4 Distribution of Labor and Classroom Community

The distribution of responsibility for learning mathematics in the classroom takes three forms: Individual learning, group learning, and whole class learning. Although the individual learning format of classroom organization normally allows for individualizing the pace and style of learning, it may generate inequities that arise from the limited opportunities of social and linguistic interactions among students, thus limiting socialization of students in the classroom. In the absence of such a process, students in the same class may learn or develop at different rates, depending on their own personal characteristics, social background, or cultural background. Consequently, these developmental differences may result in differences in engagement in learning mathematics as well as in mathematics achievement.

There are three formats for grouping students in the classroom for learning purposes. In ability grouping, the distribution of responsibility of learning mathematics, which is done on the basis of a measure of ability, results in a class structure which often corresponds to the social stratification in the school social community, thus enhancing the perception that the school perpetuates the existing social class stratification. In most cases low ability corresponds to low social class (Kutscher and Linchevski, 2000; Boaler, 1997). Moreover, homogeneous ability grouping does not encourage scaffolding in mathematics learning because of the lack of interaction among students of different ability levels. Thus, ability grouping maintains, and probably reinforces the inequitable access to mathematics learning between different social and cultural groups. Heterogeneous mixed grouping, whether collaborative or not, does not seem to pose the kind of equity issues presented by ability grouping.

In the whole class format, the primary responsibility rests with the teacher, and this may produce inequities. The very fact that the teacher addresses the perceived virtual 'average' student renders instruction, and hence the opportunity to learn, inequitable since it does not respond to the needs of individual students nor to the multiplicity of social and cultural grouping in the mathematics classroom. The participation of students is limited to answering questions or less frequently asking questions and does not provide opportunities for social and linguistic interactions among students.

In summary, the heterogeneous grouping seems to be a more favorable format for equity than ability grouping or whole class formats. This is because heterogeneous grouping allows for socialization and scaffolding, which are two processes that promote cooperation among socially and culturally different students.

4.4 Inequities Related to Student, Classroom, and Mathematics Achievement Interactions

In the activity system of mathematics education at the school level, all the processes in the system are geared towards the object of the activity, which is the achievement of the learning of mathematics. From the perspective of both the activity system and the social-cultural perspective of education, the differences in achievement associated with student factors such as gender are not by themselves inequities in achievement but rather indicators of differences in the social-cultural-pedagogic environment that accounts for such differences. Admittedly, accounting for achievement differences among students is an extremely difficult task because of the complexity of interactions of the mediating factors in the teaching/learning process, which take place in the social-cultural context. On the other hand, interpreting students' achievement differences as inequities, severely limits our ability to understand the sources of such differences and hence to address them through pedagogical action in the social-cultural context. Gutierrez (2008) states this position vividly and succinctly:

> "I outline the dangers in maintaining an achievement-gap focus. These dangers include offering little more than a static picture of inequities, supporting deficit thinking and negative narratives about students of color and working-class students, perpetuating the myth that this problem (and therefore solution) is a technical one, and promoting a narrow definition of learning and equity." p. 357

This section will present an overview of inequities in mathematics achievement associated with student characteristics (gender, socioeconomic background, and cultural background) as well as classroom characteristics. It will describe the findings from studies that have identified achievement difference and attempted to explain such difference in social-cultural-pedagogic terms.

4.4.1 Gender and Mathematics Achievement

Evidence from national, regional, and international studies indicates that, in the last two decades, gender-related differences favoring males have almost disappeared in lower grades but persisted, in more or less diminished form, towards the end of secondary school. TIMSS (2000) reported that the results of the 1995 Third International Mathematics and Science Study showed few gender differences in average mathematics achievement at the 4th and 8th grade levels, whereas in the final year of secondary school, data showed that males had significantly greater achievement than females in mathematics literacy. Data from TIMSS 2003 confirmed that the gender-related differences in grades 4 and 8 balanced out and that in some countries, mostly developed countries, females outperformed males. McGraw, Lubienski, and Strutchens (2006) reported that gender mathematics achievement gaps in the U.S National Assessment of Educational Progress (NAEP) were generally small but had not diminished across reporting years. Ma (2008) examined the evidence regarding gender differences in mathematics achievement from the latest five regional and international student assessment studies and confirmed that the general trend is that gender-related mathematics achievement differences, in favor of males, were small and that, in some cases, the differences reversed in favor of females, interestingly in some developing countries.

The diminishing gender differences in mathematics achievement over time affirm that the gender issue in mathematics achievement is a social-cultural-pedagogical one. Changes in curricula, teaching, teachers, and gender stereotypes have contributed, over time, to a reduction in gender-related differences in math achievement. Hence the focus of research related to gender shifted to classroom factors such as teachers' beliefs (Watson and DeGeest, 2005), classroom practices and organization as well as assessment tools and contexts (Leder, 2004).

4.4.2 Student Socioeconomic Background and Mathematics Achievement

Before 2000, research on the relationship between student socioeconomic status (SES) and mathematics achievement had used correlational techniques between global measures of student SES and mathematics achievement. In general, such studies found a positive correlation between the student's SES and mathematics achievement. Ma and Kishor (1997) conducted a meta-analysis of 143 studies which included, among other things, the relationship between family support and mathematics achievement. Their conclusion was that there was a significant relationship between family support and mathematics achievement and that this relationship did not interact with gender, grade level, or ethnicity. Ma and Klinger (2000), using hierarchical modeling, reported that socioeconomic status was a significant predictor of mathematics achievement. However, a recent study by Marks (2006), using data from the 2000 Program for International Student Assessment (PISA), investigated the extent to which between-school and within-school differences in mathematics, science, and reading can be accounted for by the students' SES and home resources. He concluded that difference in student performance cannot be accounted for by socioeconomic background only.

Useful as they may be, correlational studies that addressed the relation of student's socioeconomic background factors to mathematics achievement, have serious limitations in informing research, policy, or practice regarding the implications of inequities in mathematics performance. First, these studies were not often couched within a theoretical framework and hence do not adequately explain the mediating effect of SES on student learning. Second, such studies differed widely in their definitions of SES and often used global quantitative rather qualitative measures of SES based on economic and sometimes sociological considerations. Third, these studies, in their conception and design, did not take note of the complexity of the social-cultural-pedagogic context of learning. In the next paragraph, I present examples of studies which addressed inequities in mathematics performance due to student's socioeconomic background from a social-cultural-pedagogic perspective.

Using Bourdieu's concept of habitus, Zevenbergen (2001) presented evidence that low socioeconomic class students have lower achievement than middle class students because the home linguistic habitus of the latter group is more congruous with the mathematics classroom linguistic habitus. Kahn (2005) reported that, in South Africa, a policy of requiring an African language (used as a proxy to ethnicity) alongside mathematics was adopted, with the intent of reinforcing cultural identity. However, the policy resulted in socioeconomic inequity in that students who did not take an African language alongside mathematics mostly ended up attending elite schools that charge high fees. These schools have normally had better mathematics performance.

Part II of this book (Chapter 8), presents the results of an analysis to determine the impact of student level variables derived from TIMSS 2003 student background questionnaires on mathematics achievement as measured by TIMSS 2003 mathematics test scores. Among the student factors that impacted mathematics achievement and acted as inequity factors, three SES-related student factors were identified as possible inequity factors:

1. Level of parental education (in 16 of the 18 countries in the sample)
2. Student educational aspiration relative to parental education (14 countries)
3. Computer use at home (10 countries)

The student SES seems to correlate positively with mathematics achievement. However, the SES achievement gap is too complex to be interpreted in terms of social class only. The interactions of many factors in the classroom, the school, and the broader sociocultural context of the school have to be kept in mind in making inferences from studies that dealt with achievement differences associated with social class.

4.4.3 Student Cultural Background and Mathematics Achievement

The study of the relationship of the student's cultural background to mathematics achievement had been the goal of cross-cultural research since the early 1980s. A landmark in this regard was the study conducted by Stevenson, Lee, and Stigler (1986) to compare the mathematics achievement of American, Japanese, and Chinese children and account for differences in terms of 'cultural factors', such as mothers' attitudes and beliefs about their children and mathematics. In the 1990s, international large scale comparative studies started to provide cross-cultural mathematics achievement data. In general, these studies used the 'nation' as a proxy for culture. For example, achievement differences between American and Japanese students were accounted for in terms of differences between the American and Japanese 'cultures'. These studies aimed at understanding the 'cultural' factors that contributed to higher mathematics achievement in one culture in order to find ways to enhance that achievement in another.

Another line of research has focused on culture-related mathematics achievement differences associated with different cultural groups in multicultural nations such as the United States (differences between blacks and whites or hispanics and whites). With globalization and increased immigration, research started to focus on comparing the mathematics achievement of immigrants and natives. In these studies, ethnicity, color, and race were used as proxies for culture. In other cases, language grouping was used as a proxy for culture. Recently, the historical relationship of a person to a nation was used as a proxy for culture (indigenous, native, immigrant). It is extremely difficult, if not impossible, to generalize results from these studies beyond the specific definitions, designs, and tools used in a specific study because of the lack of a theoretical framework. Moreover, most of these studies failed to account for the complexity of the social-cultural-pedagogic context of learning mathematics. A third category of studies that attempted to study culture-related differences in mathematics achievement used culture as a theoretical construct. One of the most often-used constructs is Bourdieu's concept of habitus (concrete embodiment of culture in the form of thoughts,actions, and behaviors) and the related concept of cultural capital. Using these constructs, researchers in mathematics education attempted to study the extent to which various cultural groups differ in cultural capital and educational resources and the role of these in mathematics achievement disparities (Rosccingo & Ainnswerth-Darnell, 1999). Other studies used such constructs from a critical point of view to analyze and critique policies and practices from a cultural viewpoint (Kahn, 2005; Zevenbergen, 2001). A number of studies attempted interventions based on this theoretical perspective to remedy inequities in mathematical achievement. Boaler (2002) presented data from two schools, in which teachers used reform-oriented mathematics curricula, to achieve a reduction in linguistic, ethnic and class inequities in their schools. In an intervention study, Gutstein (2003) reported that students, in an urban Latino classroom who were using the NCTM Standards-based curriculum were able to understand complex issues involving justice and to develop mathematical power as a result of their involvement in real-world projects.

4.4.4 Student Perceptions of Self in Relation to the Class Community and Mathematics Achievement

Previous sections of this chapter discussed the inequities that may result from the interactions between student attributes (personal traits, socioeconomic background, cultural background) and the attributes of the mediating artifacts (physical, symbolic). Often, the perception of students and teachers of an inequity factor has a more critical role than the factor itself. Studies by Povey and Boylan (1998) and Frempong (1998, 2005) showed that, in general, students' attitudes towards engagement in mathematics at the social level is critical to the reduction of inequalities in mathematics achievement.

Part II of this book (Chapter 8), presents the results of an analysis conducted to determine the impact of student level variables derived from TIMSS 2003 student background questionnaires on mathematics achievement as measured by TIMSS 2003 mathematics test scores. The results indicate that students' perceptions of self in relation to school-related factors had a differential impact on student achievement and hence may act as potential inequity factors (For details refer to Chapter 8 of this book). The following student perceptions of self in relation to school community were found to act as potential inequity factors in mathematics achievement:

1. Self-confidence in learning mathematics (17 out of the 18 countries in the sample)
2. Student perception of being safe in school (6 out of 18 countries)

Chapter 8 also studies the extent to which students' perceptions of mathematics classroom practices acted as inequity factors in mathematics achievement. Student perceptions of the following mathematics classroom practices were found to act as potential inequity factors in mathematics achievement:

1. Students explaining their own answers (11 out of the 18 countries in the sample)
2. Students solving problems on their own (11 out of 18 countries)
3. Computer use in school (10 out of 18 countries)
4. Frequency of testing in mathematics classrooms (7 out of 18 countries)
5. Frequency of the use of calculators in mathematics classroom (8 out of 18 countries)
6. Working together in small groups (8 out of 18 countries)

4.4.5 Classroom Practices and Mathematics Achievement

The impact of student grouping in the classroom on mathematics achievement has received attention in the literature. A review of the the literature on ability grouping and tracking (Mills, 1998) reported that there were (1) no positive long-term effects for low-ability students placed in low-grouped classes; (2) positive effects for average-achieving students placed in high-track classes; and (3) no negative effects for high-achieving students in computation or problem -solving achievement, regardless of their placement. However, Kutscher and Linchevski (2000) reported dissatisfaction with ability grouping on the part of low and middle-achieving students. Burris, Heubert, and Levin (2006) reported that heterogeneous grouping leads to better mathematics participation and achievement for students from minority groups, low socioeconomic status, and all ability groups.

Teacher practices and their relation to achievement were issues that were addressed by research. Boaler (2002)reported from two studies in which teachers used reform-oriented mathematics curricula that teaching and learning practices used by the teachers were central to the reduction in linguistic, ethnic, and class inequalities in achievement. Pianta et al. (2008) who studied the impact of the quality of emotional and instructional interactions and amount of exposure to mathematics activities on trajectories of achievement in mathematics (among other things) reported that growth in mathematics achievement showed small positive correlations with observed emotional interactions and with exposure to mathematics activities.

Part II of this book (Chapter 9), presents the results of an analysis conducted to determine the impact of teacher level variables derived from TIMSS 2003 teacher background questionnaires on math achievement as measured by TIMSS 2003 mathematics test scores. The impact of each variable, which was defined and measured as the proportion of between-class variance in math achievement accounted for by that variable, served also as a measure of inequity between classes in math achievement due to this factor. The higher the proportion of between-class variance in math achievement, associated with a factor, the more the likelihood that this factor may act as an inequity factor. The results show that two factors which relate to the social dimension of the classroom account for a significant proportion of between-class variance in math achievement and hence are potential inequity factors. The two factors are: (1) Teachers' perception of school climate;and, (2) limitations on instruction due to student factors.

4.5 Inequities Related to School Policies and Sociocultural Context

This section focuses on the impact of 'rules' (school policies, social conventions, and cultural norms) on the classroom community in the activity system of mathematics education at the school level.

School policies are the explicit rules that govern student behavior in the classroom in relation to peers and teachers and to the use of mediating artifacts, as well as to the classroom organization and interactions. There is not much research on the impact of school policies on equity in mathematics education because school policies are part and parcel of the educational policies at the country level. However, depending on their intentions and nature, local school policies may, directly or indirectly, produce or limit inequities. Bartholomew (2004) gave an example of the possible impact of school policies on inequities in the mathematics classroom. He studied the case of two London secondary school mathematics departments. One adopted a policy aimed at equity and the other school did not adopt any such policy. Bartholomew concluded that the equity policy in said school, though it improved equity, produced some unwanted side effects in terms of limiting the possibilities of students to be responsible for their own learning. On the other hand, in the second school, compared to the first school, students had more opportunities for learning, yet there were greater inequalities between them. Unlike school policies whose impact on the student and the classroom can be fairly easy to identify, the impact of implicit rules represented by social conventions and cultural norms on the student and classroom is likely to be stronger than school policies and much more difficult to identify.

4.6 Concluding Remarks

The construct of the activity system seems to provide an adequate lens to organize and synthesize equity research in mathematics education at the school level. First, it has provided a sociocultural perspective for framing equity issues, which by their nature are socially and culturally constituted. Second, it has captured the complexity and interdependence of inequities in mathematics education at the school level. Third, the conception of inequities as interactions of the activity system's factors and their attributes renders inequities amenable to change through developing the relevant policies and/or practices.

The review and analysis of the relevant research in this chapter indicate that the sociocultural milieu of the school's broader community is the most powerful source of inequities in math education at the school level. The interaction of the sociocultural student background, a product of the school's sociocultural milieu, with the symbolic tools of language of instruction and of mathematics, is likely to produce inequities in engagement in math learning. On the other hand, the interactions of the students' sociocultural backgrounds with the classroom's constituency, organization, and division of labor, are likely to produce inequities in the type and degree of participation in classroom mathematics learning.

Although the school is constrained by the policies of the national education system, it has, nevertheless, a role in addressing the inequities in math education at the classroom level, where most of these inequities occur. Although math teachers may be able to deal with some inequities that arise in the classroom, they cannot, however, on their own, transform the system to be more equitable. System transformation requires basic changes in the relations among the nodes of the activity system.

The activity system suggests a general approach for transforming math education in order to address the inequities in the school. Engeström (1999) introduced the model of the expansive cycle in work teams. In the case of the school, the expansive cycle starts from some dissatisfaction with equity provisions on the part of math teachers as well as the school administration and staff. Change starts at the level of the individual teacher, through the process of internalization in which the teachers are exposed to awareness and training activities related to their perceptions of the inequities they are experiencing in their classes. As individual teachers start to apply their internalized skills and attitudes, they will engage in a process of externalization by which they try to optimize the use of their appropriated knowledge in solving specific equity problems that may arise. The successful orchestration of emerging individual teacher practices constitutes an expansive cycle which is supposed to transform the school system into a more equitable one.

5

The National Context

The activity system at the national level is linked to the school activity system by a nested hierarchical relationship. In fact, the school activity system itself is nested within the national system and acts as 'subject' in it. This inclusive hierarchical relationship between the two systems implies that the national system affects the school system and is affected by it, though to a lesser degree. As in the school activity system, the object of the math education activity in the national context is the learning of math. However, in the national system, 'school' plays the role of 'subject' (compared to 'student' in the school system) within the community of the schools of a country (compared to 'school community').

This chapter includes two major themes. First, the activity system of mathematics education in the national context will be described and its factors (nodes of the activity system) and their attributes, that may contribute to inequities in math education at the national level, will be identified. Second, the relevant research will be reviewed, synthesized, and interpreted within the framework of the activity system.

5.1 Math Education System at the National Level: Factors and Their Attributes

Figure 5.1 represents a schematic diagram of the activity system of math education at the national level. In this figure, each of the six nodes and its attributes are shown in a rectangle, with the name of the node in italics and its attributes as a list. The names of the factors (nodes) are the result of my interpretation of the factors of the activity system. The attributes that belong to each of the six nodes of the activity system are derived by logical analysis based on their relevance to equity.

Following is a brief description, with examples, of three of the factors and their relevant attributes as they apply in the activity system of mathemat-

M. Jurdak, *Toward Equity in Quality in Mathematics Education*,
DOI 10.1007/978-1-4419-0558-1_5,

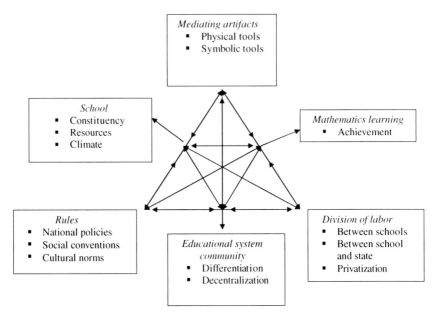

Fig. 5.1. Activity system of mathematics education at the national level with the potential inequity factors identified

ics education at the national level. The description of math learning, math mediating artifacts, and rules are the same as those in Chapter 4.

5.1.1 School

In the school as an activity system, school assumes the role of 'subject'. In fact, the students, math teachers and supervisors all constitute the 'subject' in the activity system. One of the salient school attributes is its constituency in terms of the students' sociocultural backgrounds and their personal traits, such as ethnicity, gender, and native language. Of course, we assume that the schools in one nation have, more or less, comparable variations in students' abilities and attitudes.

School resources refer to human resources as well as learning/teaching resources available to math instruction. They include teachers and their qualifications, as well as physical resources such as textbooks, calculators, computers... According to TIMSS 2003 (see Chapter 7 in this book), school climate involves three dimensions. The first dimension includes teachers' perceptions of job satisfaction, their understanding of the school's curricular goals, their success in implementing the school's curriculum, and their expectations for student achievement. A second component of the school climate is parent's support for student achievement and their involvement in school activities. A third component of school climate is students' regard for school property and their desire to do well in school.

5.1.2 Educational System Community

The educational system community consists of the students and math education community in the entire national education system. One aspect of the structure of the educational system is the degree of institutional differentiation in the system. Normally, the education system mandates institutional differentiation which requires students to choose a program or a curriculum at a certain age and this limits students' choice of programs and curricula and supposedly affects their opportunities for further education and career choices. Mathematics performance plays a role in channeling students to science or humanities programs of study and hence contributes to potential inequities produced by institutional differentiation.

Decentralization of schools allows for different degrees of school autonomy to enable schools to manage their own affairs. Many equity issues relate to school autonomy and these depend on the goals and extent of decentralization. Inequities in math education, as in any other school subject, are affected by decentralization in terms of source allocation and extent of state oversight.

5.1.3 Division of Labor

This refers to the way both labor and power are divided among the members of the educational system community, especially between the state and schools. Inequities may result from the imbalance in admission and assessment policies between private and public schools. Inequities also may result from the differences in autonomy granted to schools in the same country.

5.2 Interactions and Inequities: An Example

Inequities among schools in mathematics education at the national level are potentially generated by the interactions of the attributes of the factors in the activity system. Figure 5.1 (the bidirectional arrows in indicate such interactions), identifies the salient factors that belong to the six nodes of the activity system and their attributes. These, by themselves, are neutral to equity or inequity; it is the interactions of these factors and their attributes that may render them inequitable. The interactions of such factors or their attributes shall be called *inequity factors*.

The following example shows how interactions between the attributes of the factors in the system result in inequities in math education. For the sake of contrast two schools in a developing country are considered: One is private and the other is public. The constituency of the public school is likely to be from a predominantly low socioeconomic level and that of the private school from middle and high socioeconomic levels. It is likely that the public school students have home environments that are less favorable to learning than those of the private school students. It is also likely that the private school, in comparison to the public school, will have more and better teaching and learning resources, more qualified teachers, and more autonomy in their instructional decisions than the public school. Hence, it is reasonable to expect that the inequities in the two schools will result in different levels of math learning and achievement.

The rest of this chapter will be organized under the following titles:

1. Inequities Related to School, Education School System, and Mediating Artifacts Interactions
2. Inequities Related to the Interaction of School and Mathematics Learning Outcomes
3. Inequities Related to the Interaction of State Policies and the Education System

5.3 Inequities Related to School, Education School System, and Mediating Artifacts Interactions

5.3.1 General Pattern of Interactions

The interactions among the three factors of school, math mediating artifacts, and the educational system seem to account for most of the inequities in math education at the national level. Each of these three factors has at least one attribute which impacts the other attributes of the factor and hence defines it. Before discussing the interactions between the three factors, we shall identify and describe the defining attribute of each.

For the school factor, the school constituency is a defining attribute. First, the socioeconomic and cultural backgrounds of the students and teachers of the school define its sociocultural identity. Second, the school constituency also determines, in a direct and significant way, the quantity and quality of human and material resources available for mathematics instruction and learning in the school. Third, the two attributes of school constituency and resources together contribute towards defining the school climate.

The language used in teaching math is a defining attribute of the mediating artifacts. The language is both an artifact for communication and for cultural transmission. As a communication system, the language of instruction and learning affects the use of all other physical artifacts which use language, such as textbooks, the computer, and the internet. Language also plays a critical role in communicating mathematical concepts.

The structure of the education system is a defining factor of the educational system community. The degree of centralization and differentiation are two critical attributes of the education system structure. The degree of centralization in the system defines the extent to which schools are autonomous in their instructional decisions. On the other hand, institutional differentiation regulates the flow of students in the different curricula and programs.

How do the interactions among the defining attributes of the school, math mediating artifacts, and the educational system account for most of the inequities in math education at the national level? One can think of many patterns of interactions. One plausible such pattern is presented here. The interaction of school constituency with the use of a foreign language for math instruction is likely to produce inequities in the engagement and achievement of math learning because of the differences in home use and knowledge of that language among different socioeconomic and cultural groups. Moreover, some school cultural constituencies may regard teaching mathematics in a foreign language as discriminatory because it may carry cultural values and practices that may be incompatible with their own. Furthermore, the socioeconomic level of school constituency affects the extent to which schools can acquire and appropriate human and physical resources needed for mathematics instruction. The interaction of the school constituency with the education system is likely to produce inequities in math education. Schools with low socioeconomic level students normally depend on the government for their funding and hence have to follow a centralized system of education, which does not allow such a school autonomy in managing its own affairs. On the other hand, schools with high socioeconomic level students tend to be tuition based and consequently afford more flexibility and autonomy. Admittedly, the interactions outlined do affect inequities in other school subjects, However, with the exception of science, mathematics is more sensitive to language-related interactions than other subjects because it is more closely related to language and logic than other subjects. The complex interactions outlined often lead to a two-tier schooling system in the same country. Schools in the higher tier are perceived as having a higher degree of educational quality and as being privileged in terms of constituency and human and material resources, whereas schools in the lower tier are often perceived as having lower educational quality, and as being disadvantaged in their constituency and human and material resources. The two-tier schooling system is likely to produce two levels of mathematical literacy in the same country; one that prepares college-bound students and the other that prepares students for technical education or for the work force. The two-tier school system, being inequitable, often locks the schools in two separate modes of development (apartheid), hence maintaining, and often increasing, the gap between schools that belong to different tiers in the system.

The two-tier schooling system has historically taken different forms in different countries and is still present in almost all countries in one form or another. I believe that the factors which lead to the two-tier system differ from one country to another depending on the country's history, socioeconomic status, and social structure. The next two subsections describe and analyze two typical models of the two-tier national schooling system; one is typical of developing countries and the other of developed countries.

5.3.2 The Two-Tier Education System in Developing Countries

The so-called developing countries emerged as independent states in the few decades after the Second World War. According to Jurdak (1989), a first priority for most of these countries was to nationalize their education systems by using the national language as the language of instruction instead of the foreign languages of the colonial powers. The second priority for the newly independent states was to supply educational provisions for the increasing number of students entering the new national system of education and hence those countries had to adopt policies for universal elementary education. They also needed to educate and prepare the human resources necessary for staffing the administrations in the newly fledgling states. Third, aware of their socioeconomic disadvantage, compared to their former colonial rulers, the newly independent states started to address their lag in socioeconomic development by accelerating their development through education, science, and technology. Often, these countries looked up to their former colonial powers, to whom they were linked by ties of educational and cultural interactions, for models and sources for their own development. Fourth, these countries viewed mathematics as a subject that was the gateway to socioeconomic development and at the same time as a neutral universal subject that was not likely to affect their culture (Jurdak, 1989).

Profile of the School in the Public Sector

The urgency and challenges of meeting the educational demands of the newly independent developing states led them to adopt public education systems modeled after those of their former colonial powers, each country adapting the system to its national needs to varying degrees. This, the newly independent states generally did without much regard for the suitability of the foreign systems to the realities of their own countries. Typically, the public education system accommodated the great majority of students in the country, knowing that the system had already been strained for lack of human and material resources. Until then, the constituencies of public schools in most of these countries came from a low socioeconomic class; that itself often constituted the majority of the population. Moreover, the schools themselves suffered from poor resources, including poorly prepared teachers-a situation which generated an unfavorable climate for learning.

In public schools, the language of instruction, including that of mathematics, is the native language in most cases. In many of these cases, the equivalents of mathematical terms (which represent mathematical concepts) are translated from a foreign language into the native language without much consideration for the experiential linguistic level of students. This contributes to the students' perception of mathematics a 'technical' subject detached from experiential meaning. State-mandated mathematics textbooks, which are typically local language versions of western books, strengthen the perception that mathematics is learned by rote learning, mainly for the academic purpose of advancement in the educational system.

In most cases the public schools, which operate within a centralized system controlled by the ministry of education, have little autonomy in their instructional decisions, and hence do not have the ability to respond adequately to individual student needs. Moreover, often, the educational system limits the opportunities for choice, particularly for socioeconomically disadvantaged students, because of institutional differentiation policies that channel students to tracks within the school. Mathematics performance constitutes a key factor in the differentiation process, thus compounding the discriminatory role of institutional differentiation, especially if the system requires differentiation at an early age.

Profile of the School in the Private Sector

In general, the colonial powers kept their cultural links with the countries they had ruled through the private school system. The private schools, established during or after colonial rule, were initiated by religious missionaries, or by non-governmental, non-profit organizations, or lately, by individuals or even business firms. The current private schools are tuition-based and cater to the relatively small socioeconomically advantaged class who have had, or aspire to have, cultural ties with the societies of the former colonial power that once ruled the country. Because the constituencies of private schools in most of those countries come from the middle and upper socioeconomic classes, the schools very often have adequate resources, including well-prepared teachers in a foreign language and in mathematics and its pedagogy. Both the constituencies and resources of the private schools make the climate favorable to learning.

In some countries, the language of instruction of mathematics is a foreign language and the textbooks are imported books or locally-authored books in a foreign language. Teaching in a foreign language raises different sorts of problems. The foreign language is a cultural carrier in terms of behaviors, social relations, habits, and values (Jurdak, 1989). Some countries which are multilingual, like South Africa, resort to more than one language in teaching mathematics. In some other countries, which are multicultural, like Lebanon, schools in the private sector have competing cultural identities and use more than one foreign language. In such cases, not only is the cultural impact of the language of instruction compounded, but its social impact becomes an issue. If mathematics is taught in a foreign language, then instead of one filter, we end up with a double filter (Jurdak, 1989). Moreover, if the division between schools which use a foreign language or the native language in math instruction coincides with cultural and social class divisions, the language of instruction in mathematics will be a threat to social cohesion.

In most cases the private schools are not bound by the rigid bureaucracy of the ministries of education and as such they have more flexibility in managing their human and material resources and more autonomy in their instructional decisions. Moreover, private schools are able to work around institutional differentiation policies by enabling students to work in accordance with foreign curricula that are less stringent in their differentiation policies.

Contrasting Inequities Between Public and Private Schools

As indicated in Section 5.3.1, inequities in mathematics education result from the interactions of school constituency, language of instruction, and the education system structure. Since these three attributes differ in the public and private schools in developing countries, their patterns of interactions are likely to be different. The different patterns of interactions result in between-school inequities.

The constituency of a school reflects the choices of the community it serves and its socioeconomic and cultural identity. It is a result of parents' decisions to send their children to a particular school and this decision depends on many factors such as school proximity to home, ability to provide for school expenses, parents' perception of the school cultural identity as concretely reflected in the language of instruction of mathematics and sciences, and their perception of the quality of education in the school. Once parents choose a particular school for their children's education, any inequity that might affect the education of those children becomes a consequence of that choice. Public schools, in comparison to private schools, are perceived to offer less learning opportunities, less quality of material and human resources- especially teachers, a less favorable school climate, less school autonomy in accommodating students' learning needs, and less flexibility in manoeuvering around rigid state-mandated rules of differentiation.

How do these inequities between the public and private education systems impact mathematics education? Obviously, mathematics education is impacted in the same way other school subjects are; however, the impact of these inequities is more accentuated as far as mathematics education is concerned because of the cultural and social effects of the language of instruction in mathematics. The language of instruction in mathematics is a proxy to social class and to cultural differences. In the case of public schools in the developing countries, the translation of technical terms to the native language from a foreign language in teaching and in the textbooks contributes to the conception of mathematics as a set of definitions of mathematical terms and procedures for manipulating meaningless symbols. On the other hand, the use of a foreign language as a language of instruction in private schools may act as a divisive cultural and social factor at the national level.

5.3.3 The Two-Tier Education System in Developed Countries

The two-tier education system in developed countries has historically evolved for reasons different from those that contributed to the formation of the two-tier system in the developing countries. To illustrate the two-tier education system in the developed countries, consider two models: One from countries like the United States of America, Canada, and Australia, and the other from Western Europe. The first category of countries came into being in the last few centuries and was formed by European immigrants who championed conquering the new territories and valued the opportunities that the new land provided. Until the last few decades, those countries had valued and cherished equality as a basic tenant of their existence, but had interpreted equality as being applicable to the dominant group and not to other minorities and indigenous people in the country. In the last few decades, the model of separate development was abandoned formally but continued to exist as an undercurrent in one form or another. Although the education system in such countries seems to be unified as an equal opportunity public education system, it still has a subsystem in which educational inequities exist. We shall call this subsystem *minority public schools.*

The second category of countries consists of those old Western European former colonial powers whose economic opportunities attracted, over the last half of the past century, a massive movement of emigration from their former colonies. The immigrants sought a better life, mostly in the countries of their former rulers and were encouraged by common cultural ties such as language, and attracted by the demand of those countries for labor. The immigrants, who had cultures different from those of the people in the countries where they had settled, formed minority communities that tried to preserve their cultural identities. These communities had access to the public education system, but nevertheless, formed a de facto undeclared subsystem of the public education system in the country concerned. This subsystem is similar to the aforementioned *minority public schools*, in spite of the fact that the historical reasons for its formation are different from those of the USA model of minority public schools.

Profile of the Public School

In general, the public education system (including all undeclared sub-systems) in countries belonging to the aforementioned models is the largest and the most inclusive educational system in those countries. In such countries, the right to free compulsory pre-university education is protected by law. In those countries, school constituency typically represents the socioeconomic mix in the vicinity of the school, and as such, the middle class normally constitutes the majority in it. Instructional and learning resources are normally adequately provided and oversight by the district or state educational authorities provides a sustainable favorable environment for teaching and learning. With the exception of the minority public education system, which will be discussed in the next section, the use of the national language as a language of instruction does not normally present a pedagogical problem or cultural dissonance. However, there is variation in the developed countries in the degree of autonomy given to schools. For example, the West European countries have traditionally more centralized public education systems than the USA. In general, schools in the public education systems have enough autonomy to be responsive to the learning needs of their students.

The public education system in the developed countries does not necessarily generate systematic inequities in mathematics education. This is the case so long as there is no dominant ethnic, social, or cultural group which tries, by design or by default, to impose its culture or practices on other groups. The next section discusses minority public schools, where dissonance and conflict may arise.

Profile of the Minority Public School

The minority public schools are an integral part of the public education system in developed countries and the term is used simply to refer to those public schools which serve a predominantly minority community in such a country. The defining attribute of the minority public schools is their student constituency, which normally comes from predominantly minority students such as immigrant citizens in Europe or an ethnic group in a North American country. Resources available to minority public schools do not differ from those available to other public schools. In fact, in some countries some minority public school are given extra resources by the government to help them catch up with other schools.

The interaction of the constituency of minority public schools with the language of instruction in mathematics has a direct impact on mathematics education. The minority students in these schools (such as Latinos in the USA or North Africans in France) are learners of a second language, which is the mandated language of instruction of mathematics. One would expect that mathematics education in these schools would have pedagogical and cultural disadvantages similar to those in the multilingual and multicultural schools reviewed in Chapter 4, such as the difficulties students may face in negotiating meaning and hence in effective participation in the mathematics classroom. Cultural alienation may be another disadvantage. These disadvantages may impact negatively the opportunities of minority public school graduates for admission to higher education or access to professional fields.

In summary, it seems that the the two-tier system exists in both developing and developed countries but in different forms. In developing countries, the two-tier system consists of the public and private education systems. The two tiers in the developed countries are the the public education system and the minority public schools. The two-tier systems in the developed and developing countries differ in terms of their history and nature. However, the school constituency and the language of instruction of mathematics seem to account for most of the differences and subsequent inequities in the the educational systems of both developed and developing countries.

5.4 Inequities Related to the Interaction of School and Mathematics Learning Outcomes

5.4.1 School Socioeconomic Cultural Background and Mathematics Achievement

The focus of this section is to identify issues related to inequities in mathematics achievement between schools by reviewing a sample of studies which attempted to account for between-school differences in mathematics achievement in terms of school parameters (school composition, resources, and climate). It is to be noted that the mainstream mathematics education journals rarely addressed the issue of the relationship between differences in mathematics achievement at the school level and school parameters. Resources used will be mainly from school effectiveness research journals.

More than any school parameter, the socioeconomic school composition as it relates to school mathematics achievement has received the greatest attention in the literature. In its report on school factors related to quality and equity, PISA (2005) states that 'school composition has by far the the greatest impact on student performance' p. 45. Research on the impact of school composition on performance in mathematics education does not seem to be conclusive in that regard. In a study conducted in a socioeconomically diverse school district in Canada, Ma and Klinger (2000) report that, among other things, socioeconomic school differences are critical in explaining school differences in mathematics achievement. Opdenakkar et al. (2002) reported that class composition was very important for the explanation of between-school differences in mathematics education. Marks (2006), using the 2000 PISA data, studied the extent to which the between school differences in student performance can be attributed to students' socioeconomic background and concluded that differences in student performance in mathematics (among other things) cannot be accounted for by students' socioeconomic background. Hook, Bishop, and Hook (2007) studied the mathematics performance of students in the 'Key Standard' mathematics program, which was transplanted from the curricula of six leading TIMSS math countries, to some California districts whose cultural and economic backgrounds differ from the six TIMSS countries, but nevertheless are mostly economically disadvantaged. The authors report that performance of the students in the 'Key Standard' program was significantly superior to similar control districts. It was argued that it is rather the curriculum and the textbooks that make a difference and not necessarily the economic and cultural background of students.

5.4.2 Other School Factors and Mathematics Achievement

There is also evidence to indicate that the school climate may explain school differences in mathematics achievement (Ma & Klinger, 2000) and Opdenakkar et al., 2002). Part II of this book (Chapter 9) presents the results of an analysis to determine the impact of school level variables derived from TIMSS 2003 principal background questionnaires on between-school mathematics achievement as measured by TIMSS 2003 mathematics test scores. The impact of each variable, which was defined and measured as the proportion of between-school variance in mathematics achievement accounted for by that variable, served also as a measure of inequity between schools in mathematics achievement due to this factor. The school factors that impacted school mathematics achievement and acted as inequity factors include:

1. Principal's perception of school climate (13 out of the 18 countries in the sample)
2. Good school attendance by the students (9 out of 18 countries)

5.5 Inequities Related to the Interaction of State Policies and the Education System

The 'rules' that impact mathematics education in the activity system at the national level are the socioeconomic and cultural factors that exist in the national society as a whole as well as the state policies. Since the former factors were addressed in a previous section, this section concentrates on state policies.

State policies directly impact the attributes of the education system and consequently may be a source of inequity in mathematics education. The degree of centralization in the education system and the location and intensity of mandatory differentiation in the education system are such attributes.

5.5.1 Decentralization of the Education System and Mathematics Achievement

Decentralization of the education system has been addressed from different perspectives. Some have linked the recent decentralization of educational systems to global pressure on countries by funding agencies to promote more democratic political systems and/or to adopt market driven economies. From the perspective of democratization, the decentralization of educational system is supposed to increase school autonomy. From the perspective of free economy, decentralization is perceived as a proxy for the privatization of education.

Few studies, if any, have attempted to study the direct differential effect of the degree of decentralization on mathematics education. In fact the studies that investigated this effect often used mathematics performance as one of many criteria of the effectiveness of this education. For example, Bankov et al. (2006), using TIMSS 2003 data, investigated the effect of a decentralized implementation of a common national curriculum on the level of variation of mathematics proficiency (a measure of equity) in Bulgaria. In the same vein, Darling-Hammond et al. (2003) examined the impact of a reform project which focused on consolidating and centralizing fragmented programs and resources in a San Diego district whose schools had traditionally had an established culture of decentralization. Using mathematics performance as one of many school achievement criteria, they reported that this reform benefited the lowest-achieving schools and benefited less the most bureaucratically organized schools.

Other issues related to decentralization have been addressed. Astiz et al. (2002), conducted a quantitative analysis of data on governance and classroom implementation of eighth-grade mathematics curricula in 39 countries to demonstrate the way economic and institutional globalization have produced mixes of decentralized and centralized educational administration. In the same vein and from a critical perspective, Desmond (2002), focusing on the role of the World Bank in promoting privatization and decentralization, stated that the latter will grant more decision-making to parents and communities, but will reduce the power of the national government and national teacher unions, while ensuring employers an education most useful to their demands. PISA (2005) reported that on average across OECD countries, students in schools with more autonomy perform better in reading literacy than schools with less autonomy. One would hypothesize that the same is true for mathematics performance.

Critics of decentralization of education systems present arguments of the possible negative effects of school autonomy on school education, including mathematics education. One of those arguments is that school autonomy may have negative effects on equity, in the sense that schools will enjoy more freedom in their decisions regarding students and resources which, in the absence of close oversight of a regulatory body such as the government, may lead to inequitable access to education. Another argument is that school autonomy will put extra burden on the school administration, increasing the principal's administrative responsibilities at the expense of educational concerns.

5.5.2 Differentiation of the Education System and Mathematics Achievement

Educational differentiation may occur at the level of the classroom or at the level of the education system. The former has been discussed in Chapter 4 under the theme of student grouping. This section will focus on differentiation in the education system. This differentiation may take one of two forms: (a) Curricular differentiation i.e, channeling students at a certain grade level or age to a curriculum or (b) institutional differentiation i.e channeling students to another specialized institution.

There is hardly any study or discussion of the impact of educational differentiation at the national education system level in mainstream mathematics education journals. This is probably because differentiation is not mathematics-specific since it impacts all school subjects alike. According to

PISA (2005), the research findings indicate that system-wise educational differentiation suggests that education systems with the lowest degree of differentiation have the highest student performance level.

5.5.3 School Privatization and Mathematics Achievement

In the last two decades, privatization of education has taken new meaning. The fall of the Soviet Union has energized an international globalization movement which championed democratization at the political level and free market at the economic level. Democratization reflected itself in education systems in the decentralization of decision-making in schools and in some cases allowing schools to be semi-private, with partial support from the government in exchange for more autonomy in its decision making. In the last two decades, a few countries moved to fully privatize their schools and allow them to compete for students in the market under close government oversight.

Privatization of education may have serious implications for equity in education, including mathematics education. Since privatization follows free market laws, schools try to attract students who can afford the tuition and for that purpose they gear their marketing strategies towards promoting international education, on the assumption that the later will be more valued in the global economy. One of the claims of privatization of education is that, like privatization in economic ventures, it promotes quality improvement through competition. However, if privatization of education is allowed to operate fully according to free market rules, it will engender inequities by creating a divide between the public system and private schools. The public education system, which accommodates the great majority of students, becomes at a disadvantage in providing resources for the bulk of students it serves compared to government-independent schools that can capitalize on the resources of the economically advantaged few. Moreover, privatization may encourage the establishment of schools that serve certain cultural or religious groups having exclusionary practices that may threaten national cohesion.

5.6 Concluding Remarks

Inequities in mathematics education result from complex interactions among the components of the activity system of mathematics education at the national level. This chapter attempted to identify the main interactions and to describe the ways in which they generate system inequities in mathematics education.

The interactions of the school, language of instruction of math, and the structure of the education system are likely to produce many inequities in the opportunities to learn mathematics. In general, these interactions produce inequities which reflect themselves in a two-tier education system, which exists in both developing and developed countries but in different forms.

The differential effect of the interactions of school factors is reflected in between-school differences in math achievement. Specifically, the socioeconomic and cultural student composition of the school accounts, more than any other factor for inequities in mathematics performance. Other school factors which may lead to inequitable mathematics education performance are school climate and school resources.

The structure of the education system is also likely to generate inequities in mathematics education. The factors of school autonomy and curricular and institutional differentiation seem to be important in this regard. However, there is not enough research to support a conclusion regarding their effect in generating inequities in mathematic education.

The activity system suggests a general approach for transforming the math education school activity system in order to address the inequities in the school. The model of expansive cycle in work teams suggested by Engeström (1999) provides a vision of how to transform the national education system to be more equitable in educational provisions and math achievement. The transformation process of the system towards more equity starts with dissatisfaction with equity provisions on the part of decision makers, school principals and math teachers. The commitment to achieving the equity in quality goal has to be translated to awareness and training initiative to target those concerned at all levels. The change starts at the level of the school and math teachers as described in Chapter 4. The process will expand beyond individual schools to reach the decision-makers who have to internalize the input from schools and externalize it in the form of new policies. The successful orchestration of the emerging school experiences and practices constitutes an expansive cycle which transforms the equity practices of the system of math education at the national level.

6

The Global Context

The country math education activity system links to the global activity system by playing the role of 'subject' in the latter. However, the hierarchical relationship between the two systems is not strong because it is not based on authority as is the case between the country and the school. This results in a socially loose activity system at the global level.

This chapter deals with inequities in math education at the global level. First, the activity system of mathematics education at the global level will be described and its factors and their attributes identified. Second, the inequities that result from the interactions of those factors and their attributes will be discussed in the light of relevant literature.

6.1 Math Education System at the Global Level: Factors and Their Attributes

A schematic diagram of the activity system of math education at the national level is presented in Figure 6.1. Each of the six nodes and its attributes are shown in a rectangle, with the name of the node in italics and its attributes as a list. The names of the factors (nodes) are the result of my interpretation of the factors of the activity system at the global level. The attributes that belong to each of the six nodes of the activity system are derived by logical analysis based on their relevance to equity.

The activity system of math education at the global level differs from both the school and national systems in many respects as can be inferred from the the factors and their attributes in Figure 6.1. In the next paragraphs, the factors and their attributes will be described and exemplified.

6.1.1 Math Education

The object of the activity system at the global level is engagement in math education by the math education communities of different countries in two

M. Jurdak, *Toward Equity in Quality in Mathematics Education*,
DOI 10.1007/978-1-4419-0558-1_6,
© Springer Science+Business Media, LLC 2009

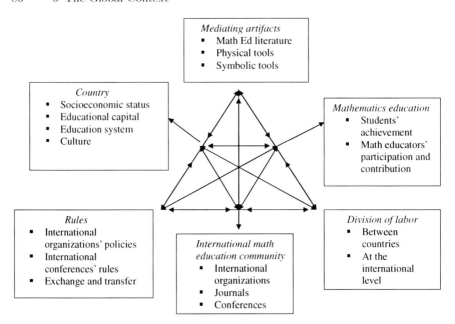

Fig. 6.1. Factors and their attributes in the activity system of mathematics education at the global level

related activities: Math learning and math education research. The countries' *achievement* of the desirable math learning outcomes constitutes the outcome of teaching and learning mathematics. On the other hand, the *participation* of math education communities in generating knowledge about math education is the outcome of engagement in research in math education.

6.1.2 Country

Research has shown that some of a country's attributes are critical for education in general, and for math education in particular. One significant attribute is the *country's socioeconomic status*, which represents the country's wealth and the way it is distributed among the population. The Gross Domestic Product (GDP) and the Gross National Index (GNI) are the best known measures of economic status for a country. Several social indicators are also used, such as Gender Parity Index. Another attribute is the *country's education capital* defined in terms of the spread of basic education as measured by the adult literacy rate as well as the level of education in the country as measured by enrollment rates at the secondary and tertiary levels. The nature of a *country's education system*, being closely related to its political system and its history, is a third attribute. Last, but not least, the *country's culture* is reflected in the ideological, social, and technological aspects of society and these impact math education. The identity of the country's mathematics education community is not only shaped by these factors but also by their interaction. For example, a country in which socioeconomic divisions coincide with cultural divisions in society would be different from one whose socioeconomic and cultural divisions do not coincide.

6.1.3 The Math Mediating Artifacts

The math mediating artifacts consist of symbolic and physical tools used by the country's education community in the teaching and learning of mathematics as well as research tools in mathematics education. The mediating tools used in the teaching and learning of mathematics were mentioned in earlier chapters and include symbolic tools such as the natural language, the language of mathematics, and physical tools such as textbooks and computers. Math education constructs, the accumulated math education literature, and ICT technologies such as the internet, are the essential tools for conducting research in math education.

6.1.4 The International Math Education Community

In principle, the international math education community consist of math educators and researchers in all countries. Compared to school and national communities, the international community has limited means for interaction. Math education international organizations, journals and conferences are the most important venues for interaction within the international community.

6.1.5 Division of Labor

Division of labor at the international level includes the division of responsibilities and power among the international math education community. The division of labor takes the form of regional cooperation in order to further math education and research in the countries of the region. Division of labor at the international level is normally done by the international organizations, which set up policies and mechanisms for assigning the responsibilities of planning and executing international activities among the different countries.

6.1.6 Rules

The rules that govern the relationships between a country's math education community and the international math education community are the policies set by the international math education organizations, editorial boards of journals, and conferences' organizing bodies. However, there are other implicit and undeclared rules stemming from rules based on political and economic power considerations.

6.2 Interactions and Inequities: An Example

The factors and their attributes are, in principle, neutral by themselves as far as equity or inequity are concerned. Inequities are generated as a result of interaction of these factors and their attributes. The interactions of such factors will be called *inequity factors*.

Using a hypothetical example, we illustrate how the interactions of the factors and their attributes generate inequities in the international activity system. Consider the math education communities in two countries, one being a developing country (low socioeconomic status) and the other a developed country (high socioeconomic status). It is likely that the math education community in the developing country does not have as much access or ownership of internet or knowledge of English as in the developed country. This by itself might generate an inequity between the two countries in terms of ownership of two mediating artifacts basic to math education. This will generate a chain reaction which results in inequitable participation of the two countries in math education at the international level. For example, because of their limited English proficiency and access to internet, the math education researchers in the developing country are at a disadvantage in communicating with the international community. Even if a math educator in the developing country succeeds in submitting a proposal to an international conference, it may not be accepted on the basis of inadequate 'quality' or questionable 'relevance' to the international community. If against all odds, a submission is accepted, its author will not have the financial resources to travel in order to participate in the conference. Obviously, this interaction of a country's socioeconomic status with the mediating artifacts (English and math education literature) may eventually lead to its exclusion from participating in math education at the international level.

The chapter will be organized under the following titles:

1. Inequities Related to Country, Community, and Division of Labor Interactions
2. Inequities Related to the Interaction of Country and Mathematics Learning
3. Inequities Related to the Interaction of International Policies and Participation

6.3 Inequities Related to Country, Community, and Division of Labor Interactions

The inequities in mathematics education at the global level may result from complex interactions among the triad consisting of country, international mathematics education community, and the division of labor. Many of the inequities in mathematics education among countries may be accounted for in terms of the country's socioeconomic economic status and culture which are likely to impact the educational capital in the country in terms of the spread and level of education in it. In general, a country with high socioeconomic level is likely to have more educational capital, and better resources for math instruction, than does a country of lower socioeconomic level. The country's socioeconomic status is critical in availing funds for research and travel, thus affecting mathematics education research productivity, which in turn, affects the country's participation in international conferences and contribution to international research journals. The country's culture also affects its participation in international mathematics education. As the English language has become the language of international conferences and journals, lack of competency in that language prevents math education researchers from participating in such conferences or publishing in such journals.

The division of labor in mathematics education among countries is determined, to a large extent, by the country's clout in research productivity. Needless to say that the less developed countries are at a disadvantage in this respect and this may lead to their partial or total exclusion from involvement in organizing international activities. These considerations give rise to a two-tier system of mathematics education at the global level: The upper tier, which we call the *optimal mode of development* in mathematics, consisting of the developed countries who participate actively in the international mathematics education community and the lower tier, which we call the *separate mode of development* consisting of the the marginalized countries who shy away from engaging actively in international activities in mathematics education.

In the last half of the past century, the decline of colonization was a major reason for the two-tiered system of mathematics education. During the age of colonization, the two-tier system did not exist because colonized countries, mostly developing countries, adopted the mathematics education of the colonial rulers. However, as colonization started to be dismantled, the developing countries, had to invest most of their resources in providing public education to increasing numbers of students. This was often done at the expense of the quality of education and of educational research and development. Hence most of the developing countries did not have the chance to accumulate enough 'credentials' in mathematics education to fully participate in the international mathematics education community.

6.4 Inequities Related to the Interaction of Country and Mathematics Learning

International comparative studies consistently indicate that the country's socioeconomic status correlates positively with the average national math achievement score. In TIMSS, for example, all developed countries are at about or above the international average in mathematics achievement while the developing countries are mostly below the international average. In Chapter 11, a set of measures of socioeconomic indicators are correlated with the national average mathematics score in TIMSS 2003. Among a number of economic indices, the Gross Domestic Product (GDP) and the Gross National Index (GNI) per capita were the two variables that correlated positively with the national mathematics achievement score. The impact on mathematics achievement, as measured by the percentage of variance in mathematics achievement accounted for, was 14% for GDP and 19% for GNI. The Poverty Rate (PR) correlated negatively with mathematics achievement and it accounted for 27% of the variance in mathematics achievement. All in all, the higher the income per capita in a country the higher the mathematics achievement and conversely the higher the PR in a country the lower the mathematics achievement.

Also in Chapter 11, the relationship between the educational capital in a country and its mathematics achievement score in TIMSS 2003 is studied. The educational capital of a country depends on the literacy rate and enrolment rate beyond basic education. Tertiary enrolment rate accounted for 37% of the variance in mathematics achievement, and adult literacy accounts for 40% of the variance in mathematics achievement.

Accounting for mathematics achievement differences among countries in terms of cultural differences is too complex to analyze. Stevenson, Lee, and Stigler (1986) pioneered studies which attempted to account for mathematics and reading achievement differences among American, Japanese and Chinese children, not only in terms of educational input but also in terms of cultural differences. The authors concluded that the cognitive abilities of the children in the three countries were similar, but large differences existed in the children's life in school (for example time spent on academic activities), the attitudes and beliefs of their mothers (the belief regarding the relative importance of the child's ability or effort in success at school), and the involvement of parents and children in school work. The authors implied an association between the lag in mathematics achievement of American children, in comparison to Japanese and Chinese children, and the differences in cultural practices and beliefs in the three countries. The much debated 'learning gap' between the USA and other developed countries, as reflected in TIMSS studies, led to the question, much debated in the USA, whether educational policies and practices can overcome cultural effects. Stigler and Hiebert (1999) addressed this question in their book *The Teaching Gap* arguing that, while it is impossible to change the culture of the the society as a whole, it is possible to change the classroom culture by making use of the best ideas from the world's teachers.

Language is a factor that may affect mathematics achievement differentially, at least in comparative international studies. The tests used in such studies are translated to the language of the country; however, much is lost, and much cultural load is carried, in such translations. Another cultural factor which may have a differential impact on between-countries mathematics achievement is the over inculcation of ideologies. The effect of this ideological factor on mathematics education is two-fold: First, such ideologies are normally taught through rote learning methods which transfer to the teaching of mathematics, and second, the instructional time given to such valued ideologies, being commensurate with its value to the society, may take away from the instructional time allotted to mathematics in the curriculum (Jurdak, 1989).

6.5 Inequities Related to the Interaction of International Policies and Participation

The interaction of international policies and regulations impacts mostly the relationship of the country with the international mathematics community and with the division of labor among the different countries. This interaction produces inequitable participation of countries in the international mathematics education community.

6.5.1 International Policies

Policies, which govern the international mathematics education institutions may result in inequities in the countries' representation on the policy-making bodies as well as their participation in international activities. As an example, we consider the International Commission on Mathematics Instruction (ICMI), which is the mother of all math education organizations and which sponsors the International Congress on Mathematics Education (ICME). ICMI is under the umbrella of the International Mathematics Union (IMU), whose membership (70 out of 195 countries in 2008) constitutes that of ICMI; the latter, however, can co-opt other member states upon the approval of the IMU executive committee (see IMU at(www.mathunion.org) and ICMI at(www.mathunion.org/ICMI)). At present ICMI, the highest international mathematics education organization, has only 72 countries represented which is less than 40% of the number of existing countries. The reason for this is that the basis for membership in IMU, and consequently membership in ICMI, *depends on the number of publications of the country in mathematics.* Most of the developing countries do not meet the criterion to join IMU and consequently ICMI. This means that countries that do not meet the criterion to join IMU lose their opportunity to join ICMI's membership, simply because they are not active in mathematics research, in spite of the fact that they may be very active in mathematics education.

The obstacles that face math educators from developing countries when attempting to participate in international conferences are many and varied. Some of those obstacles relate to the policies and practices of the organizing bodies of these conferences and some to the countries themselves. Normally, international conferences are organized in developed countries in cities that have the infrastructure and specialized human resources to support such large conferences. For math educators of developing countries, the cost of attending such conferences can be daunting, as there are neither resources nor traditions in their country to support their participation. However, there is increasing awareness on the part of the international mathematics education organizations of the need to alleviate some of the financial burden on mathematics educators from developing countries to enable more of them to participate in international conferences. There is also an effort to provide assistance in editing the English of their contributions.

Another policy which puts some math educators at a disadvantage with regard to their participation in international conferences is the adoption of English as the language of such conferences. Moreover the call for these conferences is usually done through emailing lists which, in most cases, are based on previous participation. Furthermore, the policies that govern acceptance of contributions do not have enough flexibility to allow a wide range of diverse profiles in content and format, though such contributions may be perceived as meaningful in the contexts of the authors' countries.

The same can be said about international journals of mathematics education. The publication policies of such journals are almost standardized along Western scientific journals and consequently exclude contributions that address local issues perceived by their authors as meaningful in both the local and the international contexts. Because of the stringent standards in refereed journals, the English language is more of a barrier in international math education journals than it is in conferences.

6.5.2 Exchange and Transfer

Exchange of mathematics education research and experiences is one way for countries to learn from one another and consequently to bridge any gap in their mathematics education development. ICMI has sponsored many regional conferences for that purpose in different regions of all continents such as:

- ICMI East Asia Regional Conferences on Mathematics Education
- Espace mathematique
- All-Russian Conference on Mathematical Education
- Inter-American Conferences on Mathematics Education
- First Africa Regional Conference

Another form of one-way exchange is the transfer of the mathematics education experiences of one country to another. One motivation for such transfer is that some developing countries look up to more influential countries because the latter are perceived to be superior politically, economically, or educationally. The transfer of USA NCTM Standards to many countries is an example of such extensive transfer. Recently, curricula and textbooks of countries which consistently ranked highly in international assessment studies, like Singapore, started to be transferred to other countries, such as the USA. However, if not adapted to the cultural and social conditions of the receiving country, the transfer of mathematics education from one country to another may result in possible exclusionary practices of some social or cultural groups.

6.6 Concluding Remarks

The inequities in mathematics education at the global level are the result of complex interactions among the triad consisting of country, international mathematics education community, and the division of labor. The defining attributes of these factors seem to be the country's socioeconomic status and its culture which determine to a large extent, the country's educational capital and help shape the country's education system in terms of governance and resources for mathematics instruction.

The inequities that were generated by the interactions among factors and attributes of the system, helped create a two-tiered system of mathematics education at the global level. The upper tier, which we called *the optimal mode of development* includes the developed countries integrated in the international mathematics education community. The lower tier, which we called *the separate mode of development* consists of the marginalized countries that have yet to be integrated in the international activities in mathematics education.

The country's socioeconomic status as well as its culture have a differential effect on mathematics achievement. Data from international assessment studies indicate that the higher the income per capita in a country the higher the mathematics achievement. On the other hand, the higher the poverty rate in a country the lower the mathematics achievement. Some authors attempted to explain differences in mathematics achievement among countries in terms of between-country cultural differences, which led mathematics educators to focus on closing the learning gap through addressing the teaching gap. They recommended capitalizing on the best international teaching practices to optimize learning.

The rules that govern the functioning of the international mathematics education community produce inequities in mathematics education. These inequities are reflected in the extent to which mathematics educators participate and contribute to international conferences and journals as well as the extent to which countries are represented in international mathematics education organizations. It seems that inequities among developing and developed countries exist in both participation and representation in the international mathematics education community.

Perhaps it is easier to deal with inequities at the global level than at the school or national levels because the former is an ad hoc socially loose system that is free of national bureaucracies. The transformation of the global system may be achieved through a three-prong strategy based on Engeström model of expansive transformation (1999):

Reflection at the country level: The country's math education community identifies and reflects on the obstacles that face it in being integrated into the international math education community.

Addressing inequities at the country level: The country's national community starts to address the sources of inequities at the country level. This can take many forms depending on the country's system.

Transformation of the international system: The international organizations of math education come up with necessary policy and organizational changes in order to allow for participation of more developing countries.

Equity in Quality in Mathematics Education: Across Countries Comparisons Based on TIMSS 2003 Results

7

Methodology

7.1 A Theoretical-Methodological Issue

In Part I of this book the activity system as a theoretical model for analyzing and interpreting research on equity and quality in mathematics education was introduced. In Part II of the book, the stepwise multiple regression model was used to analyze TIMSS 2003 data and to investigate the relative differential impact of selected school-related contextual variables on mathematics achievement in order to identify those factors that contribute to inequities in mathematics education in each of the 18 countries and compare these factors across countries. It looks as if two methodologies that are conceptually incompatible are being used. Activity theory research suggests that there is a methodological discrepancy between research based on activity theory and research based on contextual theories because of conceptual differences between the two types of theories. This section explores this methodological discrepancy and attempts to rationalize the use of a hybrid methodology of the two theories in this book.

7.1.1 Research Method in Activity Theory

The activity system is grounded in Leont'ev activity theory. One core concept of activity theory is its interpretation of human individual development. According to Leont'ev (cited in Tolman, 1999), human 'development cannot be fully understood in terms of the acquisition of adaptive behaviors' p. 74. The essence of individual human development is a process of *appropriation*, defined by Leont'ev as mastering historically accumulated experience. The implication of the appropriation method is that understanding individual human development is to be done through a method compatible with the appropriation concept. This method (called the concrete research method) has to:

(1) be based on analyzing the process by which appropriation happens and not the change of the object of the activity

M. Jurdak, *Toward Equity in Quality in Mathematics Education*,
DOI 10.1007/978-1-4419-0558-1_7,
© Springer Science+Business Media, LLC 2009

(2) aim at explaining the appropriation rather than describing the surface features of actions

(3) be based on observing a behavior pattern while developing and not a fully developed one. Engeström (1987) developed the activity system in order to explain, not only individual activity, but also collective activity in which the 'subject' consists of a group, rather than one individual. The activity system, being an extension of the activity theory, strives to adhere to the basic concept of appropriation. However, it is not clear how the concrete research method of activity theory applies to the development or *transformation* of the activity system. According to Engeström (1999):

> "In order to understand such transformations going on in human activity systems, we need a methodology for studying expansive cycles. Such methodology does not easily fit into the boundaries of psychology or sociology or any other particular discipline." p. 35

Engeström further suggests "that such a methodology is best developed when researchers enter actual activity systems undergoing such a transformation" p. 35. In a way, this suggestion implies the use of the concept of appropriation and hence the use of the concrete research method.

7.1.2 Research Method in Contextualism

Developmental contextualism attempts to analyze and understand human development in the light of the multiple levels of interactions between individuals' characteristics, psychological as well as biological, and their environments. According to developmental contextualism, developmental changes are reciprocal or bidirectional relations, in the sense that the context changes the individual just as the context is changed by the individual. In contrasting society and context, Tolman (1999) considers human development in contextualism to be basically different from that of activity theory in that the former recognizes adaptive processes due only to biological maturation and experience, that result in the acquisition of new patterns of behavior. On the other hand, activity theory recognizes, in addition to maturation and experience, the process of appropriation which enables the individual to reproduce historically accumulated human capacities and functions. Research in contextualism aims at establishing and accounting for the complex interactions between the individual's factors and those of the context in which the individual is functioning. Often this method takes the form of correlational model-fitting analysis.

The use of two seemingly discrepant theoretical frameworks is a limitation which has two mitigating considerations. First, to enter the actual activity systems to study equity as it unfolds in each system, as suggested by Engeström, is not possible in this book, as 18 huge multi-layered activity systems would have to be compared and contrasted i.e the educational systems themselves. Second, the next best alternative to that is to study the interactions in the systems *at one point in their history and try to interpret the interactions from the perspective of the activity system.* TIMSS 2003 provided data on the status of mathematics performance and the national contexts in many countries including the 18 countries studied in this sample. These data provided an opportunity to explore the impact of student, teacher, and school contextual factors on math achievement and hence on equity. However, the activity system lens will be used to interpret these interactions.

7.2 TIMSS 2003 Background Questionnaires

The International Association for the Evaluation of Educational Achievement (IAE), has conducted so far four international comparative studies of student achievement in mathematics and sciences. The third TIMSS (Trends in International Mathematics and Science Study) assessed eighth-grade and fourth-grade students in both mathematics and science. This round of testing is known as TIMSS 2003. TIMSS gathered information about students' educational experiences together with their mathematics and science achievement assessment data, in order to identify factors related to math achievement. The development of TIMSS 2003 background questionnaires is described in Chrosrowski (2004) and was based on TIMSS's especially designed contextual framework. The international versions of the questionnaires are in TIMSS 2003 International Database (Martin, 2005b). The data from three types of background questionnaires were used in this study:

1. The school questionnaire asked school principals or headmasters to provide information about the school contexts for the teaching and learning of mathematics and science
2. The teacher questionnaire, completed by the mathematics and science teachers of sampled students, collected information about the teachers' preparation and professional development, their pedagogical activities, and the implemented curriculum. For the eighth grade, there were separate versions for mathematics teachers and science teachers
3. The student questionnaire, completed by eighth grade students who were tested, sought information about the students' home backgrounds and their experiences in learning mathematics and science

7.3 Summary Indices and Derived Variables from Questionnaire Data

TIMSS 2003 collected data on many hundreds of variables from the students, teachers, and principals who participated in the study. The purpose of these data is to help policymakers, curriculum specialists, researchers, and others to better understand the performance of their educational systems. In addition to the data on the original questions asked in the various questionnaires, TIMSS created a range of indices and derived variables that summarized the data. The TIMSS 2003 definitions of these indices are given in Martin (2005c).

7.3.1 Student-Level Indices

1. *Index of Time Student Spends Doing Mathematics Homework*: The index is computed from students' responses to the the two questions regarding mathematics homework: How often does your teacher give you homework in mathematics? When your teacher gives you mathematics homework, how many minutes are you usually given to do it?
2. *Index of Self-Confidence in Learning Mathematics*: The index is computed from students' responses to the following items: The extent to which the student perceives that he/she usually does well in mathematics, mathematics is easier for him/ her than for many of classmates, mathematics is one of his/her strengths, and the student perceives that he/she learns things quickly in mathematics. The higher the index the higher the self-confidence in learning mathematics.
3. *Index of Student Valuing Math*: The index is computed from students' responses to the following seven items : I would like to take more mathematics in school, I enjoy learning mathematics, I think learning mathematics will help me in my daily life, I need mathematics to learn other school subjects, I need to do well in mathematics to get into the university of my choice, I would like a job that involves using mathematics, and, I need to do well in mathematics to get the job I want. The higher the index the higher the student's valuing math.
4. *Index of Student Perception of Being Safe in School*: The index is computed from students' responses to items which measure the extent to which the student has a feeling of being safe in school (not subject to stealing, bullying, intimidation, ridicule, or neglect by other students).
5. *Index of Parents Highest Education Level*:The index is computed from students' responses which measure the highest educational level by either parent. The higher the index the higher the level of parents education.
6. *Index of Student Educational Aspirations Relative to Parents Educational Level*: The index is computed from students' responses to items which measure student's educational aspirations relative to parents' educational level. The higher the index the higher the student's educational aspirations relative to parents' educational level.
7. *Index of Computer Use*: The values of this variable are student's use of computer both at home and at school, at home but not at school, at school but not at home, only at places other than home and school, does not use computer at all.

7.3.2 Teacher-Level Indices

1. *Index of Teacher Reports on Teaching Mathematics Classes with Few or No Limitations on Instruction due to Student Factors*: The index is based on mathematics teachers' responses to limitations on instruction related to: Students with different academic abilities, students who come from a wide range of backgrounds, students with special needs, uninterested students, students with low morale, and disruptive students.

2. *Index of Teacher Emphasis on Mathematics Homework*: The index is computed based on math teachers' responses to the following questions: How often does the math teacher assign homework? On the average, how long does the student take to finish the homework?

3. *Index of Mathematics Teacher Perception of School Climate*: The index is computed from teachers' responses regarding their characterization of the the following school climate factors: Job satisfaction, understanding of the school's curricular goals, degree of success in implementing the school's curriculum, expectations for student achievement, parental support for student achievement, parental involvement in school activities, students' regard for school property, students' desire to do well in school.

4. *Index of Mathematics Teacher Perception of Safety in the Schools*: The index is computed from teachers' responses to the following items concerning security in their schools: This school is located in a safe neighborhood; I feel safe at this school; school's security policies and practices are sufficient.

5. *Class Size For Mathematics Instruction.*

6. *Math Teacher Has Full License or Certification.*

7.3.3 School-Level Indices

1. *Index of Principal Perception of School Climate*: The index is computed from principals' responses regarding their characterization of the following school climate factors: Teachers' job satisfaction, teachers' understanding of the school's curricular goals, teachers' degree of success in implementing the school's curriculum, teachers' expectations for student achievement, parental support for student achievement, parental involvement in school activities, students' regard for school property, students' desire to do well in school.

2. *Index of Good School and Class Attendance*: The index is computed from principals' responses to the frequency and severity of the following behaviors:Arriving late at school, absenteeism, skipping class.

3. *Trends in Index of Availability of School Resources for Mathematics Instruction*: The index is computed from principals' responses to questions regarding shortages or inadequacies that can affect instruction in their school: Instructional materials (e.g., textbooks), budget

for supplies (e.g., paper, pencils), school buildings and grounds, heating/cooling and lighting systems, instructional space (e.g., classrooms), computers for mathematics instruction, computer software for mathematics instruction, calculators for mathematics instruction, library materials relevant to mathematics instruction, audio-visual resources for mathematics instruction.

4. *Number Of Hours Of School Per Year*.
5. *Number Of Weeks Of School Per Year*.

7.4 Single-Item Variables

The single-item variables are scaled responses to selected items. These items were selected for this study, because they were judged to measure the perceptions of students and teachers of math classroom practices. Henceforth, these variables will be referred to as *practices*.

7.4.1 Student-Level Variables

1. How often do you speak language of TIMSS test at home?
2. How often do you explain your answers in mathematics lessons?
3. How often do you work problems on your own in mathematics lessons?
4. How often do you have a quiz or test in mathematics lessons?
5. How often do you use calculators in mathematics lessons?
6. How often do you work together in small groups in mathematics lessons?
7. How often do you listen to the teacher give a lecture-style presentation in mathematics lessons?
8. How often do you decide on your own procedures for solving complex problems in mathematics lessons?
9. How often do you relate what you are learning in mathematics to your daily life?

7.4.2 Teacher-Level Variables

1. In teaching mathematics to the students, how often do you usually ask them to work together in small groups?
2. How often do you usually assign gathering data and reporting in mathematics homework?
3. How do you use textbook(s) in teaching mathematics?
4. In teaching mathematics, how often do you usually ask students to explain their answers?
5. How often do you usually assign finding one or more applications of the content covered?
6. In teaching mathematics, how often do you usually ask students to relate what they are learning in class to their daily lives?

7. In teaching mathematics, how often do you usually ask students to decide on their own procedures for solving complex problems?

7.5 Dependent Variables

TIMSS estimates each student's achievement based on the student's responses to the items that they took and the student's background characteristics. Because there is some error inherent in this imputation process, TIMSS draws five such estimates, or 'plausible values,' for each student on each of the scales. Each student, therefore, has five estimates of his or her achievement on the TIMSS mathematics and science scales. *The Average Mathematics Plausible Score (AMPS)* defined as the average of the five plausible values for the overall mathematics achievement was used in this study as a measure of overall mathematics achievement. *The Average Plausible Score for the Mathematics Teacher (APSMT)* was computed to be the mean of the average of the mathematics plausible score for the students in the sample taught by that mathematics teacher. *The Average Plausible Score for the School (APSS)* was computed as the mean average plausible score of the students in the sample in that school.

7.6 The Sample of Countries

A sample of 18 countries were selected out of the 45 countries which participated in TIMSS 2003. The selection of the sample of countries was done using stratified random sampling by region and by population size. The 45 countries were classified into the eight UNESCO regions. The countries were also classified into three categories of population size (high, middle, low) based on their population size relative to the region they belong to. From each region, three countries of high, middle, and low population size were selected. If the region included three or less countries, all of them were included in the sample. Table 7.1 shows a breakdown of the sample of countries by region and population size.

TIMSS 2003 followed a standard sampling procedure for all countries. In each country, representative samples of students were selected using a two-stage sampling design. Although countries could, with prior approval, adapt the sampling design to local circumstances, in general, countries selected at least 150 schools at the first stage using probability-proportional-to-size sampling. At the second stage, one or two classes were randomly sampled in each school. Generally, this resulted in a sample size of at least 4,000 students per country. Some countries opted to include more schools and classes which resulted in larger sample sizes. This they did in order to be able to do additional analyses.

Table 7.1. The sample of countries by region and population size

Region	Country	Population size
• Arab States	Egypt	High
	Lebanon	Low
	Saudi Arabia	Medium
• Central and Eastern Europe	Hungary	Low
	Romania	Medium
	Russian Federation	High
• Central Asia	Armenia	Low
• East Asia and the Pacific	Australia	Medium
	Indonesia	High
	Singapore	Low
• Latin America and the Caribbean	Chile	Low
• North America and Western Europe	Italy	Medium
	Netherlands	Low
	United States	High
• South and West Asia	Iran, Islamic Rep.of	Medium
• Sub-Saharan Africa	Botswana	Low
	Ghana	Medium
	South Africa	High

7.7 Statistical Analysis

Two statistical analyses were used in this study, namely step-wise multiple regression and variance component. Step-wise multiple regression estimates the percentage of each variable which enters the regression equation independently of the other variables in the equation. Variance component analysis estimates the percentage of variance associated with a random variable. For each of the 18 countries five runs of stepwise regression were used as follows:

1. Stepwise regression with the student indices as predictors and the Average Mathematics Plausible Score (AMSP) as dependent variable
2. Stepwise regression with the student practices as predictors and the Average Mathematics Plausible Score (AMSP) as dependent variable
3. Stepwise regression with the math teacher indices as predictors and the Average Plausible Score for the Mathematics Teacher (APSMT) as dependent variable
4. Stepwise regression with the math teacher practices as predictors and the Average Plausible Score for the Mathematics Teacher (APSMT) as dependent variable
5. Stepwise regression with the school background variables, related to mathematics, as predictors and the Average Plausible Score for the School (APSS) as dependent variable

The variance component analysis was done to compare the variance accounted for by the school as a random variable. The results of this analysis were used to compare the eight Arab countries on the extent to which variance across schools account for variance in achievement.

7.8 Equity Measure

Measures of equal educational opportunity estimate the extent to which the variation in a given factor accounts for variation in an indicator of interest. For example, a measure of equal opportunity of students of different socioeconomic levels to achieve in mathematics may be estimated by the extent to which the variation in math achievement is accounted for by the variation in socioeconomic level. The higher the proportion of the variation in students' math achievement due to student socioeconomic level, the less the equity in math achievement among different socioeconomic levels. In other words, this would mean that student socioeconomic level makes a difference in math achievement.

Based on this concept of equity, we present the following definitions, which we shall be using through Part II of this book.

7.8.1 Inequity Index

The *inequity index* in math achievement is defined as the percentage of the total variance in math achievement accounted for by a specified factor, *independently of any factor in a specified set of factors*. The inequity index varies between 0 and 1. An inequity index of 0 means that the factor does not account for any variance in math achievement and hence there is almost complete equity in math achievement among the members in the group under consideration. On the other hand, an inequity index of 1 means that the factor accounts for almost all the variance in math achievement and hence there is almost no equity in math achievement among the members of the group under consideration. The larger the inequity index, the higher the inequity in math achievement, relative to that factor.

7.8.2 Inequity Factor

An inequity factor is a factor which has an inequity index significantly greater than 0. The factor may belong to a student, class, school, or country. If the inequity factor is student-related, then the inequity index refers to the percentage of the total *between-student* variance in math achievement accounted for by the specified student-related factors. The inequity index for class, school, or country factors is similarly defined.

8

Student-Related Inequity Factors

This chapter focuses on identifying and investigating student-related inequity factors in mathematics achievement, based on *TIMSS 2003 Student Background Questionnaire* and TIMSS 2003 assessment data. According to our definition, a student-related inequity factor is one that accounts for a significant percentage of between student-variance in mathematics achievement. For each of the 18 countries in the sample, two runs of stepwise multiple regression were done, one with the student indices as predictors, and another with the student single-item variables as predictors (will henceforth be referred to as practices). In both cases, the Average Mathematics Plausible Score (AMPS) was used as a dependent variable (Section 7.5).

The stepwise multiple regression results are presented in a uniform pattern. An inequity factor, whether index or practice, is included in the discussion in this chapter, if it satisfies two conditions. First, the inequity factor should be significant, i.e. it should account for a significant (> 0) percentage of variance in (AMPS). Second, the inequity factor should be significant in at least six of the 18 countries in the sample. For each inequity factor that satisfies the two conditions, we present a figure consisting of a two-part bar graph:

1. Sub-figure (a) represents the the inequity factor's strength (percentage of variance in the math achievement score accounted for by the inequity factor) for each country. It is used to identify the pattern of the inequity factor's strength across countries.
2. Sub-figure (b) represents the country's math average by inequity factor level for each country. It is used to identify the pattern of math mean differences associated with the levels of the inequity factor, across countries.

The theoretical framework of the activity system at the classroom/school level, whose center (subject) is the student, will be used to interpret the significant inequity factors as interactions between the nodes of the system (Chapter 3). For easy reference we reproduce here the figure representing mathematics education as an activity system at the classroom/school level, with factors and their attributes identified. The rest of this chapter will be

M. Jurdak, *Toward Equity in Quality in Mathematics Education*,
DOI 10.1007/978-1-4419-0558-1_8,
© Springer Science+Business Media, LLC 2009

divided into two sections, one on indices and the other on practices. In each section, a subsection will be allotted to each index or practice.

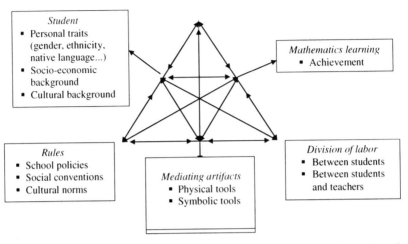

Fig. 8.1. Factors and their attributes in the activity system of mathematics education at the school level

8.1 Student Indices

For each of the 18 countries, the seven student indices were entered in a stepwise multiple regression model using student's math score as a dependent variable (see Chapter 7). The two indices, namely Index of Time Student Spends Doing Mathematics Homework and Index of Student Valuing Math, did not meet the inclusion criterion (significant in at least six countries) and hence were not presented in this chapter.

It is to be noted that all five student indices that were inequity factors are not math specific, except for student self-confidence in learning mathematics. This indicates that student attributes that impact equity in math achievement are, in general, not directly related to math, but rather to the socioeconomic-cultural background of student.

8.1.1 Index of Student Educational Aspiration Relative to Parents' Education

This index measures the level of student educational aspiration relative to parents' education. Figure 8.2 (a) shows that this index was an inequity factor in all countries in the sample, except in Egypt and the United States of America.

The percentage of between-student variance of mathematics achievement accounted for by this index ranged between 28 (Hungary) and 1.3% (Australia). An examination of the bars reveals that there is no apparent pattern in the relationship between the strength of this index and the developmental factors of the countries. For example, the group of the three countries in which this index had the highest strength (Hungary, Romania, Botswana) and the group in which the index had the least strength (Australia, Saudi Arabia, Lebanon) both include countries belonging to different regions and having different developmental indicators. What is remarkable, however, is that this index was an inequity factor in mathematics achievement in all but two countries and that its impact cuts across cultural, social, economic, and regional boundaries.

Figure 8.2 (b) shows that the higher the student educational aspiration relative to parents' education, the higher the mathematics achievement in each of the 16 countries in which this index was an inequity factor. The mean difference in mathematics achievement was most pronounced between the highest and lowest levels of educational aspiration (in favor of the former). This difference reached about 140 points (equivalent to 1.4 standard deviations of TIMSS standardized score) in countries such as in Hungary, South Africa, and Chile. It seems that the student's educational aspiration relative to parents' education is a strong inequity factor that makes a difference in math achievement.

How does student's aspiration relative to parents' educational level relate to the activity system at the classroom/school level? Referring to Figure 8.1, this index seems to belong to student personal traits, since it is a personal belief. However, a student's educational aspiration is socially constituted as a result of the interaction of the student with the home environment, on one hand, and with the classroom community, on the other. These results confirm the research trends in Chapter 3, regarding the effect of interactions of student socioeconomic-cultural home habitus and of classroom community on equity in math education.

Is student's educational aspiration amenable to change by changing classroom practices or school policies? There is little that can be done regarding the home environment in this regard. However, classroom practices may contribute to enhancing students' educational aspirations. This is because students' valuation of their education, and hence their educational aspirations, are partially formed as a result of their interaction with teacher and peers. Making the learning of math more meaningful and relevant to students may enhance students' educational aspirations.

8.1.2 Index of Student Self-confidence in Learning Mathematics

The Index of 'Self Confidence in Learning Mathematics' measures student's perception of how well he/she usually does in mathematics, whether mathematics is easier for the student than for many of classmates, whether mathematics is one of her/his strengths, and whether he/she learns things quickly in

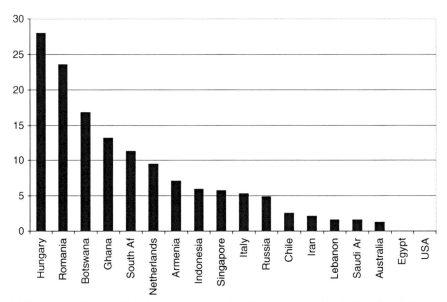

(a) Percentage of between-student variance in student math score accounted for by the index of student educational aspiration relative to parents' education, by country

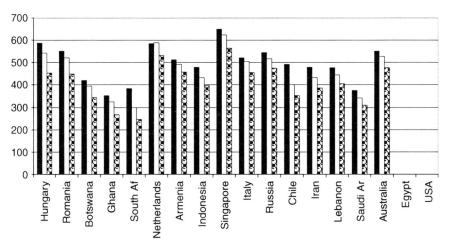

■ Student aspires to finish university and either parents went to university or equivalent
□ Student aspires to finish university but neither parent went to university or equivalent
▨ Student does not aspire to finish university regardless of parents' education

(b) National math average score by level of the index of student educational aspiration relative to parents' education, by country.

Fig. 8.2. The impact of student educational aspiration relative to parents' education on math achievement

mathematics. The higher the index the higher the self-confidence in learning mathematics.

Figure 8.3 (a) shows that this index was an inequity factor in all countries in the sample except Indonesia. The percentage of variance in mathematics achievement accounted for by this index ranged between 23.4 percentage (Australia) and 1.3% (Singapore). An examination of the bars in Figure 8.3 (a), reveals that there is no apparent pattern in the relationship between the strength of this index and the developmental factors of the countries. For example, the three countries in which this index had the highest impact (Australia, Italy, Russian Federation) are countries that are developed countries; whereas, those in which the index had the least impact (Singapore, Armenia, South Africa) had the highest TIMSS scoring country (Singapore) and the lowest scoring country (South Africa) and those two countries belong to different regions and have different developmental indicators. What is remarkable, however, is that this index was an inequity factor in all but one country, and that its impact cut across cultural, social, economic, and regional boundaries.

In each of the 17 countries in which this variable had a significant impact on mathematics achievement, Figure 8.3 (b) shows that the higher the student self confidence in learning mathematics, the higher the mathematics achievement. The mean difference in mathematics achievement was most pronounced between the highest and lowest levels of student self-confidence in learning mathematics (in favor of the former). This difference reached about 90 points (equivalent to 0.9 standard deviation of TIMSS standardized score) in Australia, for example. It seems that student self confidence in learning mathematics is a strong inequity factor that makes a difference in math achievement.

How does student self confidence in learning mathematics relate to the activity system at the classroom/school level? Referring to Figure 8.1, on the surface, this index seems to belong to student personal traits, since it is a personal belief. However, student self confidence in learning mathematics is primarily formed as a result of student's interactions with the math teacher and with classroom peers during math instruction. To a lesser degree, student self-confidence in learning mathematics is influenced by the home environment, especially parents' perceptions of value of mathematics and of their child's capacity for learning mathematics. It is highly likely that student self confidence in learning mathematics is primarily influenced by the interaction of the students with math mediating artifacts (math teacher) and to a lesser degree by social and cultural factors in the classroom and at home.

Is student self confidence in learning mathematics amenable to change by changing classroom practices or school policies? This index is math-specific, and hence the math teacher's practices are critical in enhancing student's math self-concept, and hence self-confidence in learning math. Later in this chapter, we provide evidence that practices such as giving opportunities to students to explain their answers and to solve problems on their own impact math

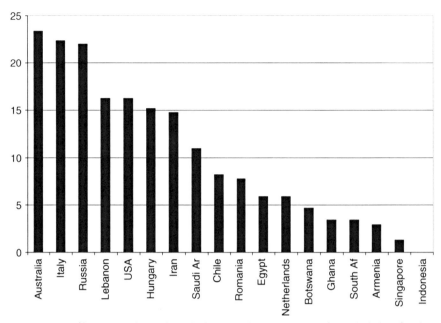

(a) Percentage of between-student variance in student math score accounted for by the index of student self-confidence in learning math, by country

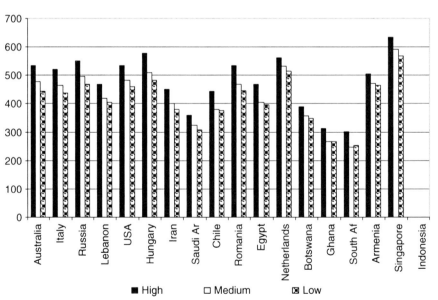

(b) National math average by level of the index of students' self-confidence in learning math, by country

Fig. 8.3. The impact of students' self-confidence in learning math on math achievement

achievement. Consequently, building students' autonomy and responsibility for learning math may enhance their confidence in learning the subject.

8.1.3 Index of Parents Highest Education Level

This index measures the highest degree by either parent. The higher the index, the higher the level of parents education. Figure 8.4 (a) shows that this index was an inequity factor in all except four countries in the sample (Armenia, Indonesia, Botswana, Russian Federation). The percentage of variance of mathematics achievement accounted for by this index ranged between 37.1 (in Chile) and 1.2% (in Italy).

An examination of the bars in Figure 8.4 (a) reveals that the group of the three countries in which this index had the highest impact (Chile, Egypt, Lebanon) are developing countries; whereas, those in which the index had the least impact (Singapore, Romania, Italy) are developed countries. However, there is no clear pattern for the countries in which parents' education had an average impact on mathematics achievement. The level of parents' education was an inequity factor in the great majority of the countries (14 out of 18), and thus its impact cut across cultural, social, economic, and regional boundaries. However, the impact of parents' education level on math achievement may be higher in developing countries than in developed countries.

Figure 8.4 (b) shows that the higher the index of parents' education level, the higher the mathematics achievement in each of the 14 countries in which this index was an inequity factor. The mean difference in mathematics achievement was most pronounced between the parents having a university degree or higher and those having no more than primary education(in favor of the former). This difference reached about 151 points (equivalent to 1.5 standard deviation of TIMSS standardized score) in Chile, for example. This shows that parents' level of education is a strong inequity factor that makes a difference in math achievement.

How does parents' educational level relate to the activity system at the classroom/school level? Referring to Figure 8.1, this index seems to belong exclusively to student socioeconomic background. Parents' educational level is outside the influence of the school and hence it is not amenable to change by changing school policies or classroom practices. However, the negative effects of parents' educational level on classroom math learning may be offset by adapting classroom practices and school policies to take into account the needs of students coming from low socioeconomic backgrounds.

8.1.4 Index of Computer Use

This index measures the extent to which students use computers and the context in which they use them. The five levels of the index are: Student uses computer both at home and at school, at home but not at school, at school

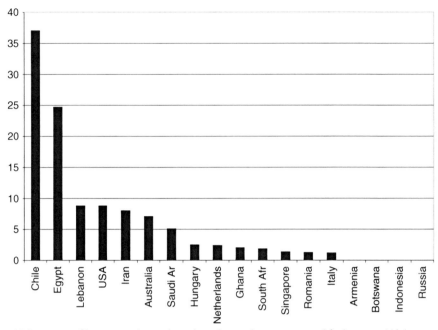

(a) Percentage of between-student variance in student math score accounted for by parents' highest education level, by country

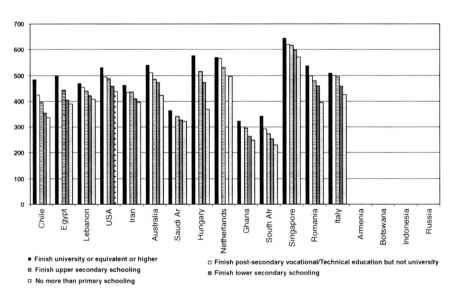

■ Finish university or equivalent or higher   □ Finish post-secondary vocational/Technical education but not university
▨ Finish upper secondary schooling   ▨ Finish lower secondary schooling
□ No more than primary schooling

(b) National math average by category of parents' highest education level, by country

Fig. 8.4. The impact of parents' highest education level on math achievement

but not at home, only at places other than home and school, does not use the computer at all.

Figure 8.5 (a) shows that this index was an inequity factor in 10 out of the 18 countries in the sample. The range of the percentage of variance of mathematics achievement accounted for by this index was small, the highest being 3.8% in Singapore and the lowest being 1.1% in Iran and Netherlands. Student use of the computer seems to have little impact on math achievement, relative to previous student indices. It is to be noted that the strength of use of the computer as an inequity factor was low, probably because of the small variance in computer use in the countries concerned.

An examination of the bars in Figure 8.5 (a) reveals that there is no apparent pattern in the relationship between the strength of this index and the developmental factors of the countries. For example, the group of the three countries in which this index had the highest strength (Singapore, Chile, Indonesia) and the group in which the index had the least strength (Netherlands, Iran, Ghana) both include countries belonging to different regions and having different developmental indicators.

Figure 8.5 (b) shows that computer use at both school and home was associated with the highest mean mathematics score for the nine of the ten countries in which this index was an inequity factor. Computer use at home but not school had the next highest mean math score in seven of the nine countries. In other words, computer use is most effective in enhancing math achievement when it takes place at both school and home.

Figure 8.1 indicates that computer use belongs to the mediating artifacts. The results indicate, however, that computer use is most effective in enhancing math achievement if it used at both home and school. The availability and computer use at home is related to the student socioeconomic background. Hence, the impact of computer use on math achievement is mediated by the student socioeconomic background. This is in line with the results of research we reviewed in Chapter 3.

8.1.5 Index of Student Perception of Being Safe in School

This index measures the extent to which the student has a feeling of being safe in school (not subject to stealing, bullying, intimidation, ridicule, or neglect by other students). Figure 8.6 (a) shows that this index was an inequity factor in only six countries out of the 18 countries in the sample. The percentage of variance of mathematics achievement accounted for by this index ranged between 7% (Lebanon) and 1.1% (Ghana). All the six countries, are known to have suffered from political and social unrest.

Figure 8.6 (b) shows that the higher the student's perception of being safe in school, the higher the mathematics achievement in each of the six countries in which this index was an inequity factor. The mean difference in mathematics achievement was most pronounced between students with high and low perception of safety (in favor of the former). This difference reached

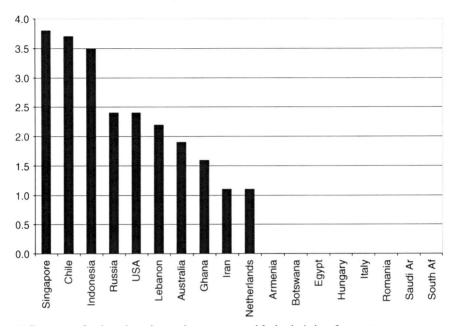

(a) Percentage of variance in student math score accounted for by the index of computer use, by country

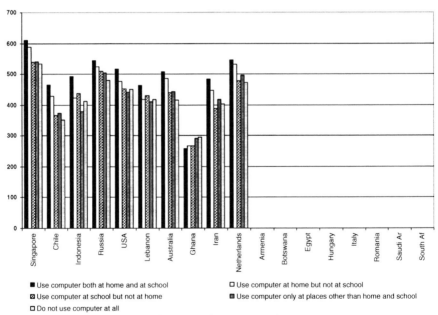

■ Use computer both at home and at school   □ Use computer at home but not at school
▨ Use computer at school but not at home   ▥ Use computer only at places other than home and school
□ Do not use computer at all

(b) National math average by level of the index of computer use, by country

Fig. 8.5. The impact of the of the student computer use on mathematics achievement

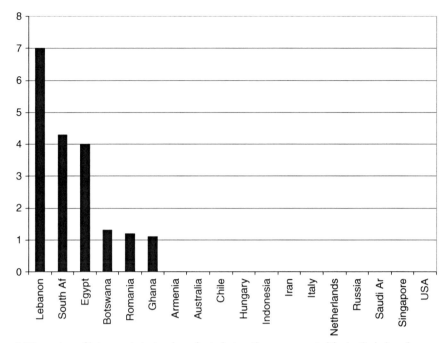

(a) Percentage of between-student variance in student math score accounted for by the index of student perception of being safe in school, by country

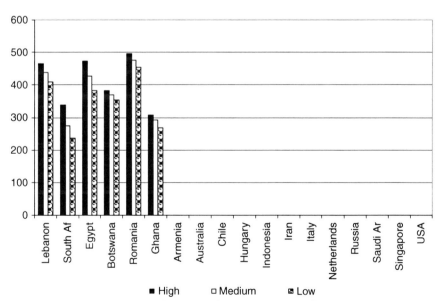

(b) National math average by level of the index of students' perception of being safe in the schools, by country

Fig. 8.6. The impact of student perception of being safe in school on math achievement

about 55 points (equivalent to 0.55 standard deviation of TIMSS standardized score) in Lebanon.

Obviously, student perception of being safe in school is related to classroom and school environments which belong to the 'rules' and 'classroom community' in the activity system at the classroom/school level (Figure 8.1). Explicit school policies and implicit norms in the school impact students' perceptions of being safe from bullying, intimidation, ridicule, or neglect by other students in the classroom and in the school. It is possible to enhance students' perception of being safe in school by examining the relevant school policies and classroom practices.

8.1.6 Summary of Student Indices as Inequity Factors

Student indices are composite measures defined by TIMSS to reflect students' perception regarding their classroom and school experiences. Out of the seven student indices defined by TIMSS 2003, three were math-specific. Two of those, namely, Index of Student Valuing Math, and Index of Time Student Spends Doing Mathematics Homework, did not meet the criterion for inclusion (significant in at least six countries) as inequity factors. The third index, namely, Index of Self-Confidence in Learning Mathematics, had the strongest impact among the five indices that qualified as inequity factors.

Table 8.1 presents a summary of the student indices which were found to be inequity factors, the strength of each (percentage of variance in math achievement accounted for by it), and the possible interactions in the classroom/school activity system, which account for the inequity attributed to each of them. Table 8.1 shows that the interactions of two or more of the following nodes (or their attributes) may account for the inequity in math achievement:

Table 8.1. Summary of student indices as inequity factors in the activity system

Inequity factor	Average strength	Interactions in the activity system that account for the inequity
▪ Index of Self-Confidence in Learning Mathematics	10.9	• Student cultural background • Math mediating artifacts
▪ Index of Student Educational Aspirations Relative to Parents Educational Level	8.8	• Classroom community • Student socioeconomic background
▪ Index of Parents Highest Education Level	8.1	• Student • Classroom community
▪ Index of Student Perception of Being Safe in School	3.2	• Rules • Classroom community
▪ Use of computer	2.4	• Math mediating artifacts • Student socioeconomic background

- Student: socioeconomic background and cultural background
- Classroom community: classroom practices
- Math mediating artifacts: teaching methodology and computers
- Rules: School policies and home cultural norms

8.2 Student Practices

Student practices are single-items in the TIMSS 2003 Student Background Questionnaire each of which elicits a response regarding the students' perception of how often a math classroom teaching/learning practice occurs. This questionnaire was examined to identify items that measure students' perception of math classroom practices. As a result we identified nine such practices (see Chapter 7 for definitions). For each of the 18 countries, the nine practices were entered in a stepwise multiple regression model using the student math score as a dependent variable. A practice was included in this chapter if it satisfied the criterion for inclusion, namely if it was a significant inequity factor in at least six countries. The four practices of speaking language of test at home, listening to the teacher give a lecture-style presentation, deciding on one's own procedures for solving complex problems, and relating what is learnt in mathematics to daily life did not meet this criterion and hence were not included in this chapter.

Although the teaching/learning practices belong to the classroom community in the activity system of math education at the classroom/school level, their formation, and students' perception of them, are the result of complex interactions of the nodes and their attributes in the activity system. For example, the practice of asking students to solve problems on their own is the result, among other things, of how authority is perceived and practiced in the school community, as well as, of what the school philosophy and culture are.

The deep-rooted causes for math classroom practices are difficult to identify, let alone to change. However, the practices themselves are under the control of the school and math teachers, and in principle, lend themselves to change through teacher professional development and change of school policies. Such changes in teaching/learning practices are not necessarily sustainable, if not accompanied by transforming the activity system as a whole.

8.2.1 How Often Students Explain Their Answers in Mathematics Lessons

Figure 8.7 (a) displays the percentage of variance in mathematics achievement accounted for by students' perception of 'how often they explain their answers in mathematics lessons'. Figure 8.7 (a) shows that this practice is an inequity factor in 11 out of the 18 countries in the sample. The percentage of variance of mathematics achievement accounted for by this practice ranged between 6.2 (in Lebanon) and 1.1% (Armenia).

There seems to be no apparent relationship between the strength of this inequity factor and the developmental status of the country in which this practice was an inequity factor. One would observe, however, that eight of the 11 countries in which this practice was an inequity factor were developing countries and scored below the international math average in TIMSS 2003.

Figure 8.7 (b) shows that the more students explain their answers in mathematics classroom, the higher the mathematics achievement. The difference in the mean mathematics score is the highest between students explaining their answers 'for every lesson' and 'never'. This difference reached 82 points (equivalent to 0.82 standard deviation of TIMSS standardized score, such as in Ghana.

The practice of asking students to explain their answers in math lessons is closely related to the perceived role of the student in math classrooms. In some ways this practice is affected by the perception of responsibility and power in the math classroom, namely the division of labor in the activity system (see Figure 8.1). This division of labor is closely related to the value system of the school community.

8.2.2 How Often Students Work Problems on Their Own in Mathematics Lessons

Figure 8.8 (a) displays the percentage of variance in mathematics achievement accounted for by students' perception of 'how often they work problems on their own in mathematics lessons'. Figure 8.8 (a) shows that this practice was an inequity factor in 11 out of the 18 countries in the sample. The percentage of variance of mathematics achievement accounted for by this variable ranged between 8.6 (Singapore) and 1% (South Africa).

Figure 8.8 (b) shows that the more students work problems on their own in class, the higher the mathematics achievement. The difference in the mean mathematics score was the highest between students working problems on their own 'for every lesson' and those 'never' doing so. For example, in Singapore this difference reached 105 points (equivalent to 1.05 standard deviation of TIMSS standardized score).

It is worth noting that Singapore, the highest math-achieving country in TIMSS 2003, was the country in which the practice of having students work problems on their own had the highest impact on mathematics achievement. It is also worth noting that the three countries (Singapore, Italy, Australia) in which this practice had the highest impact on mathematics achievement were developed countries, whereas the three countries (South Africa, Egypt, Saudi Arabia) in which this practice had the least impact were developing countries.

The practice of having students work problems on their own is one aspect of the division of labor in the math classroom community. It also reflects the dominant cultural values regarding the role of responsibility and power in mathematical discourse.

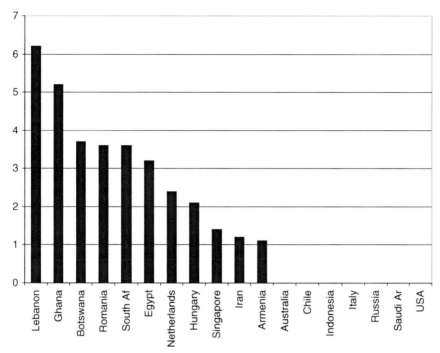

(a) Percentage of between-student variance in student math score accounted for by how often students explain their answers in mathematics lessons, by country

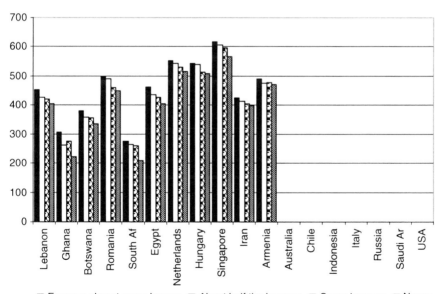

■ Every or almost every lesson   □ About half the lessons   ▨ Some lessons   ▨ Never

(b) National math average by level of how often students explain their answers in mathematics lessons, by country

Fig. 8.7. The impact of how often students explain their answers in mathematics lessons on math achievement

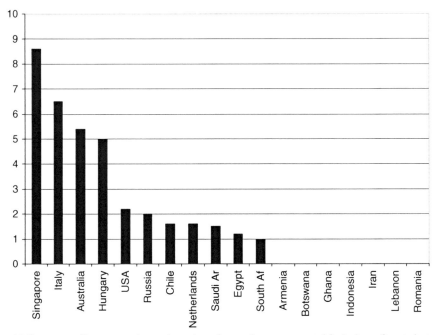

(a) Percentage of between-student variance in student math score accounted for by how often students work problems on their own in mathematics lessons, by country.

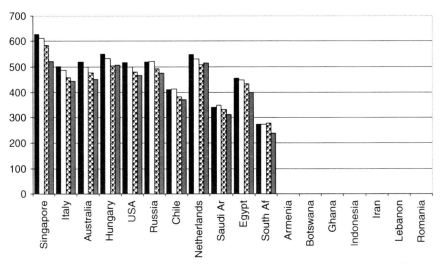

■ Every or almost every lesson □ About half the lessons ▣ Some lessons ▨ Never

(b) National math average by level of how often students work problems on their own in mathematics lessons, by by country

Fig. 8.8. The impact of how often students work problems on their own in mathematics lessons on math achievement

8.2.3 How Often Students Have a Quiz or Test in Mathematics Lessons

Figure 8.9 (a) displays the percentage of variance in mathematics achievement accounted for by students' perception of how often they have a quiz or test in mathematics lessons. The figure shows that this practice was an inequity factor in seven out of the 18 countries in the sample and that the percentage variance of mathematics achievement accounted for by this variable ranged between 4.1 (in Netherlands) and 1.1% (Saudi Arabia).

Figure 8.9 (b) shows that the highest mean mathematics achievement score was associated with the response of having a quiz or test in 'some lessons', and the lowest mean with excessive testing, namely, 'having a test or quiz in every or almost every lesson' or with no testing 'never have quiz or test'. This difference reached 91 points (equivalent to 0.91 standard deviation of TIMSS standardized score) in the United States. It seems that the moderate use of testing in mathematics classrooms is associated with higher mathematics achievement as compared to excessive testing.

Testing practices in math classroom are affected by school policies and the philosophy of the educational system. Both factors belong to the 'rules' in the activity system.

8.2.4 How Often Students Use Calculators in Mathematics Lessons

Figure 8.10 (a) displays the percentage of variance in mathematics achievement accounted for by students' perception of how often they use calculators in math lessons. This practice was an inequity factor in eight out of the 18 countries in the sample. The percentage of variance in mathematics achievement accounted for by this practice ranged between 9.5 (Saudi Arabia) and 1.3% (Botswana).

Figure 8.10 (b) shows that there are two patterns. For Singapore, the United States, and Hungary (all three countries scored above international average in TIMSS 2003), the highest mean mathematics achievement score was associated with the response of using calculators in 'every lesson' and the lowest mean mathematics achievement score was associated with 'never' using calculators. For the remaining five countries (all scored below international average), the highest mean mathematics achievement score was associated with the response of 'never' using calculators and the lowest mean mathematics achievement score was associated with 'every lesson'.

The impact of using calculators on mathematics achievement seems to be moderate and country-specific. In high achieving countries, the more frequently calculators are used, the higher the mathematics achievement, whereas in low achieving countries, the less frequently the calculators are used, the higher the mathematics achievement. Consequently, the inequities that may arise from using calculators in mathematics classrooms should be

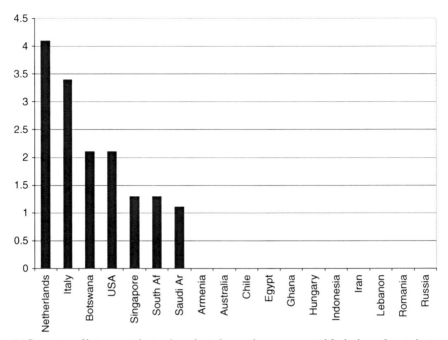

(a) Percentage of between-student variance in student math score accounted for by how often students have a quiz or test in mathematics lessons, by country

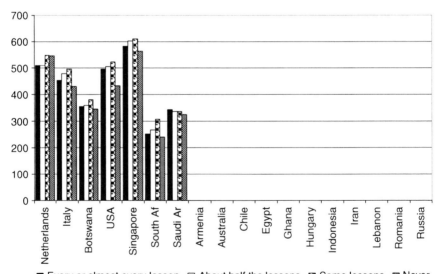

(b) National math average by level of how often students have a quiz or test in mathematics lessons, by country

Fig. 8.9. The impact of how often students have a quiz or test in mathematics lessons on math achievement

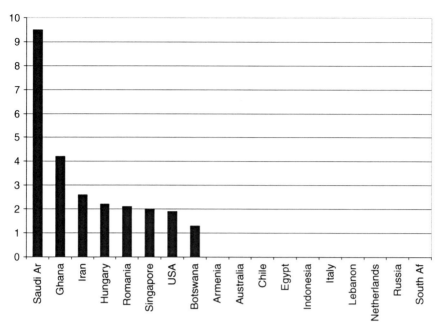

(a) Percentage of between-student variance in student math score accounted for by how often students use calculators in mathematics lessons, by country

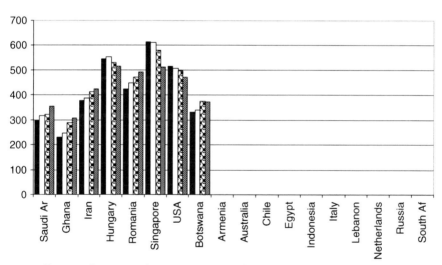

■ Every or almost every lesson ☐ About half the lessons ▨ Some lessons ▨ Never

(b) National math average by level of how often students use calculators in mathematics lessons, by country.

Fig. 8.10. The impact of how often students use calculators in mathematics lessons on math achievement

addressed according to the country in question and according to the objective and modality of using calculators in that country.

The use of calculators in the math classroom is related to a number of factors in the activity system. One factor is the availability of calculators which depends on the socioeconomic level of the school. A second factor is school policies regarding the use of calculators in school instruction and assessment. A third factor is a social-cultural factor, namely, the degree to which the use of calculators is pervasive in the social and economic life of the school community.

8.2.5 How Often Students Work Together in Small groups in Mathematics Lessons

Figure 8.11 (a) displays the percentage of variance in mathematics achievement accounted for by students' perceptions of how often they work together in small groups in mathematics lessons. The figure shows that this practice was an inequity factor in eight out of the 18 countries in the sample. The percentage of variance of mathematics achievement accounted for by this variable ranged between 8.3 (South Africa) and 1.3% (Singapore).

Figure 8.11 (b) shows that the highest mean mathematics achievement score was associated with students' responses of working together in small groups in 'some lessons' or 'never'. The lowest mean mathematics achievement score was associated with students' responses of working together in small groups in 'all lessons'. The impact of students' working together in small groups on mathematics achievement seems to be moderate. It seems that the less frequently students work together in small groups, the higher the mathematics achievement.

The practice of having students work together in small groups is closely related to school policies regarding classroom organization. On the other hand, school policies are influenced by the dominant cultural values regarding competition, cooperation, and team work.

8.2.6 Summary of Student Practices as Inequity Factors

What we called student practices refer to students' perceptions of math classroom teaching and learning practices. Out of the nine student practices, five qualified as inequity factors. The impact of those five student practices on mathematics achievement, and hence their strength as inequity factors, was much less than for student indices. This is probably because the index, by definition, is a multidimensional composite score, while the practice is a single item score.

The five practices differ in the direction of their impact on math achievement. For the two practices, namely, having students explain their own answers in math lessons and having students solve problems on their own, the more students explain their answers and solve problems on their own in math

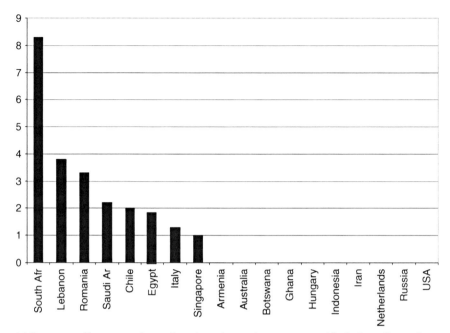

(a) Percentage of between-student variance in student math score accounted for by how often students work together in small groups in mathematics lessons, by country.

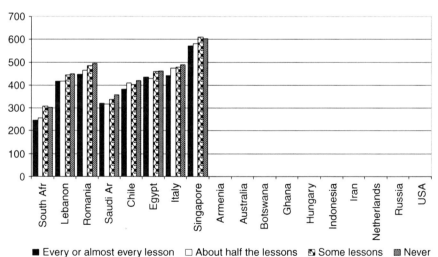

■ Every or almost every lesson   □ About half the lessons   ▨ Some lessons   ▩ Never

(b) National math average by level of how often students work together in small groups in mathematics lessons, by country

Fig. 8.11. The impact of how often students work together in small groups in mathematics lessons on math achievement

lessons, the higher the mathematics achievement. The frequency of testing in mathematics classrooms had an impact on mathematics achievement and the trend was that moderate use of testing in mathematics classrooms was associated with higher mathematics achievement, while excessive testing (almost every lesson)was associated with low math achievement.

The two practices, namely, the use of calculators in mathematics classroom, and working together in small groups seem to have a moderate impact on math achievement. However, the use of calculators is country-specific. In high achieving countries the more frequently calculators are used the higher the mathematics achievement, while in low achieving countries the less frequently the calculators are used the higher the mathematics achievement. In general, the less frequently students work together in small groups, the higher the mathematics achievement. It seems that the excessive use of this practice does not necessarily promote mathematics achievement.

Table 8.2 presents a summary of the student practices which were found to be inequity factors and the possible interactions in the classroom/school activity system, which may account for the inequity attributed to each of them. Table 8.2 shows that the interactions of two or more of the following nodes (or their attributes) may account for inequity in math achievement:

- Division of labor: Division of responsibility and power in classroom
- Classroom community: Classroom practices and organization
- Math mediating artifacts: Teaching methodology and calculators
- Rules: School policies and cultural norms

Table 8.2. Summary of student practices as inequity factors in the activity system

Inequity factor	Interactions in the activity system that account for the inequity
▪ How often students explain their own answers in math lessons	• Division of labor • School community culture (rules)
▪ How often students solve problems on their own in math lessons	• Division of labor • School community culture (rules) • Math mediating artifacts
▪ How often students use calculators in math lessons	• School socioeconomic level • School policies and culture (rules) • Math mediating artifacts
▪ How often students work together in small groups	• Classroom organization • School policies and culture (rules)
▪ How often students have a test in math lessons	• School policies • Educational system

9

Teacher-Related Inequity Factors

This chapter focuses on investigating the impact of teacher-related inequity factors based on the *TIMSS 2003 Teacher Questionnaire* and TIMSS 2003 math assessment data. In this chapter, the teacher-related factors measure teachers' perceptions of selected school and classroom practices, as much as they can be derived from *TIMSS 2003 Teacher Questionnaire*. The dependent variable is the *The Average Plausible Score for the Mathematics Teacher (APSMT)*. Since the original TIMSS teacher file did not include the mean math score of the students taught by the same teacher, a linkage program was developed to assign for each math teacher the mean math score of his/her students. The *APSMT* was computed to be the mean of the Average Mathematics Plausible Score for the students in the sample taught by that mathematics teacher (see Chapter 7). In this chapter, *a teacher-related inequity factor is defined to be a teacher-related factor that accounts for a significant percentage of the between-class variance (classes taught by the same math teacher)*.

For each of the 18 countries in the sample, two runs of stepwise multiple regression were done, one with the teacher indices as predictors and another with the teacher single variables as predictors (henceforth will be referred to as *teacher practices*. In both cases, the APSMT was used as the dependent variable.

The stepwise multiple regression results are presented in a uniform pattern. An inequity factor, whether index or practice, is included in the discussion in this chapter, if it satisfies two conditions. First, the inequity factor should be significant, i.e. it should account for a significant (> 0) percentage of variance in APSMT. Second, the inequity factor should be significant in at least six of the 18 countries in the sample. For each inequity factor that satisfies the two conditions, a figure consisting of a two-part bar graph is included:

1. Sub-figure (a) represents the the inequity factor's strength (percentage of variance in the math achievement score accounted for by the inequity factor) for each country. It is used to identify the pattern of the inequity factor's strength across countries.

M. Jurdak, *Toward Equity in Quality in Mathematics Education*,
DOI 10.1007/978-1-4419-0558-1_9,
© Springer Science+Business Media, LLC 2009

2. Sub-figure (b) represents the country's math average by inequity factor level for each country. It is used to identify the pattern of math mean differences associated with the levels of the inequity factor, across countries.

The theoretical framework of the activity system at the classroom/school level will be used to interpret the significant inequity factors as interactions between the nodes of the system (Chapter 3). The rest of this chapter will be divided into two sections, one on teacher indices and the other on teacher practices. In each section, a subsection will be allotted to each index or practice.

9.1 Teachers' Indices

For each of the 18 countries, the six teacher indices were entered in a stepwise multiple regression model using *The Average Plausible Score for the Mathematics Teacher (APSMT)* as a dependent variable (see Chapter 7). The two indices, namely Index of Mathematics Teachers' Perception of Safety in the Schools and Math Teacher Has Full License or Certification, did not meet the inclusion criterion (significant in at least six countries) and hence were not presented in this chapter.

9.1.1 Index of Mathematics Teachers' Perception of School Climate

This index is computed from teachers' responses regarding their characterization of the the following school climate factors: Job satisfaction, understanding of the school's curricular goals, degree of success in implementing the school's curriculum, expectations for student achievement, parental support for student achievement, parental involvement in school activities, students' regard for school property, and students' desire to do well in school.

Figure 9.1 (a) shows that this factor was an inequity factor in all countries in the sample except South Africa, Saudi Arabia, Lebanon, and Italy. The percentage of variance of between-class mathematics achievement accounted for by this index ranged between 23.4 (Chile) and 2.5% (Australia). The bar graph 9.1 (a) shows that out of the top seven countries, four are developed countries, whereas four of the bottom seven countries are developing countries. What is remarkable, however, is that this index was an inequity factor in all but four countries and thus its impact cut across cultural, social, economic, and regional boundaries.

Figure 9.1 (b) shows that the more positive the mathematics teachers' perception of school climate, the higher the mathematics achievement in each of the 14 countries in which this index was an inequity factor. The mean difference in class math achievement was most pronounced between the most and least positive perception of school climate (in favor of the former) and this difference reached about 105 points (equivalent to 1.05 standard deviations of TIMSS standardized score) in Chile.

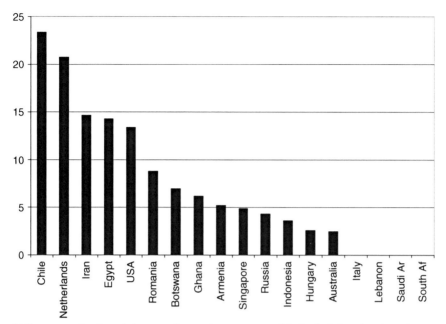

(a) Percentage of variance in between-class math score accounted for by the index of mathematics teachers' perception of school climate, by country

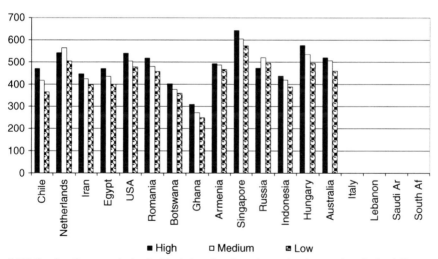

■ High   □ Medium   ▨ Low

(b) National math average by level of the index of mathematics teachers' perception of school climate, by country

Fig. 9.1. The impact of teachers' perception of school climate on mathematics achievement

How does teachers' perception of school climate relate to the activity system at the classroom/school level? Referring to Figure 8.1, this index seems to belong to the interaction of math teacher, as a member of school community, and school policies and culture, as well as, the home culture, as reflected in parental involvement and their support for their children's achievement.

Is school climate amenable to change by changing classroom practices or school policies? There is much that the school can do to improve the its climate, and hence teachers' perception of it. Through its policies and practices, the school can influence directly many of the components of school climate. For example, the school can promote teachers' understanding of the school's curricular goals, support teachers in their efforts to raise the degree of success in implementing the school's curriculum, and raise teachers' expectations for student achievement. As an employer, the school can enhance teachers' job satisfaction. Moreover, the school can work with the students to improve their regard for school property and their desire to do well in school.

9.1.2 Index of Teachers' Reports on Teaching Mathematic Classes with Few or no Limitations on Instruction due to Student Factors

This index is based on mathematics teachers' responses to limitations on instruction related to students: Having different academic abilities, coming from a wide range of backgrounds, having special needs, not interested in learning, having low morale, or being disruptive. Figure 9.2 (a) shows that this factor was an inequity factor in seven out of the 18 countries in the sample. The percentage of variance of between-class mathematics achievement accounted for by this index ranged between a remarkable 35.7% (Australia) and 3.6% (Italy). All seven countries, with the exception of Indonesia, are developed countries that scored above the international math average in TIMSS 2003.

The high variance in mathematics achievement associated with this index in those seven countries, reflects a relatively large variance in teachers' perception regarding limitations on instruction due to student factors. One plausible interpretation of this result is that those countries, which are relatively rich, can afford to provide for special needs, through differentiation of instruction. Teachers in these countries are probably aware of issues related to differentiation of instruction for special needs students. Math teachers' sensitivity may account for variation in teachers' reports regarding limitations on instruction due to student factors. On the other hand, the countries in which this index was not an inequity factor, do not have much variation in this factor because of uniform lack of instructional provisions for special needs students.

Figure 9.2 (b) shows that the more strongly (high level) the teacher perceives few or no limitations on instruction due to student factors, the higher the mathematics achievement in each of the seven countries in which this variable had a significant impact on mathematics achievement. The mean difference in mathematics achievement was most pronounced for the difference

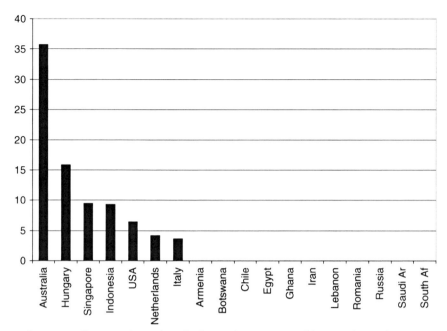

(a) Percentage of between-class variance in class math score accounted for by the index of teachers' reports on teaching mathematic classes with few or no limitations on instruction due to student factors, by country

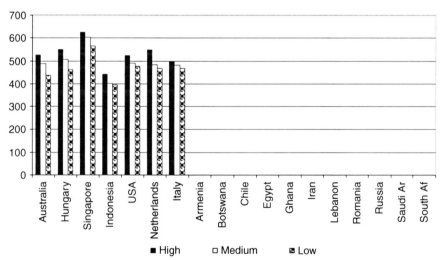

■ High   □ Medium   ▣ Low

(b) National math average by level of the index of teachers' reports on teaching mathematic classes with few or no limitations on instructions due to student factors, by country

Fig. 9.2. The impact of teachers' reports on teaching mathematic classes with few or no limitations on instructions due to student factors on mathematics achievement

between 'no or few limitations' and 'many limitations' (in favor of the former) and this difference reached about 99 points (about 0.99 standard deviations of TIMSS standardized score) in Australia. This indicates the extent to which limitations on instruction due to student factors' has on mathematics achievement.

The limitations on math instruction due to student factors are at the heart of equity for special needs students, and every student is special in her or his own way. Referring to the activity system of mathematics education at the classroom level (Figure 8.1), one can see that this index is closely related to the interaction of two nodes of the system: Student and math mediating artifacts. All student attributes (personal traits, socioeconomic and cultural backgrounds) are potential limitations on math instruction, especially when they interact with the math mediating artifacts, including math teaching methods and learning and instructional tools.

The limitations on math instruction due to student factors are amenable to change by changing math teachers' perception of these limitations and how to deal with them in the classroom through professional development. To achieve these changes, school culture and policies need to be aligned with the objective of decreasing inequity in math learning due to student factors.

9.1.3 Index of Teachers' Emphasis on Mathematics Homework

This index is computed based on math teacher's responses to whether he/she assigns homework, how often, and, on the average, how long it is supposed to take the student to finish. Figure 9.3 (a) shows that this index was an inequity factor in six out of the 18 countries in the sample. The percentage of variance of mathematics achievement accounted for by this index ranged between 6.3% (Australia) and 2.1% (United States). The bar graph in 9.3 (a) shows that five of those six countries are developed countries and scored above international average in TIMSS 2003. This means that the high variance in mathematics achievement associated with this factor in those six countries reflects a relatively larger variance in the teachers' emphasis on mathematics homework than other countries.

Figure 9.3 (b) shows that, in each of the six countries in which this index was an inequity factor, the more the emphasis on mathematics homework, the more the mathematics achievement. The mean difference in mathematics achievement was most pronounced between 'high emphasis' and 'low emphasis' on mathematics homework (in favor of the former). For example, in Hungary this difference reached about 79 points, which is 0.79 standard deviations of TIMSS standardized score.

Referring to the activity system of mathematics education at the classroom level (Figure 8.1), one can see that the emphasis on mathematics homework is mainly related to mathematics mediating artifacts. This factor is amenable to change by changing the practices of the mathematics teacher in terms of the frequency and length of mathematics homework.

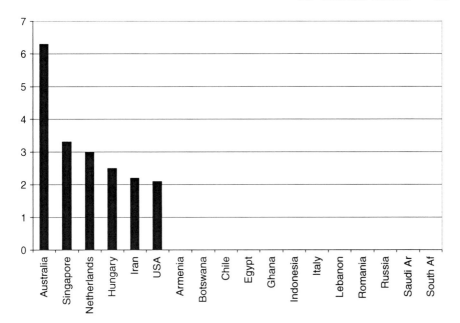

(a) Percentage of between-class variance in class math score accounted for by the the index of teachers' emphasis on mathematics homework, by country

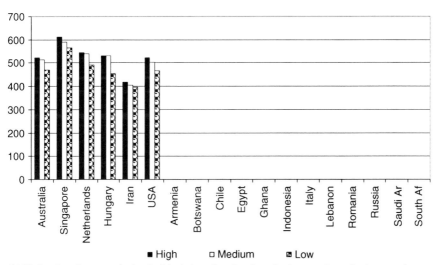

(b) National math average by level of the index of teachers' emphasis on mathematics homework, by country

Fig. 9.3. The impact of teachers' emphasis on mathematics homework on mathematics achievement

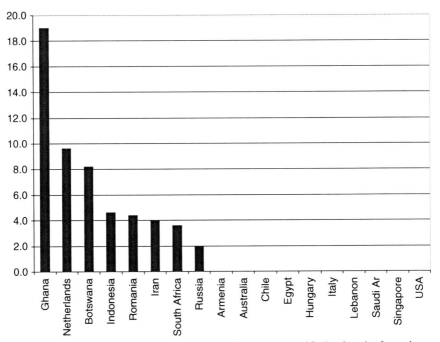

(a) Percentage of between-class variance in class math score accounted for by class size for mathematics instruction, by country

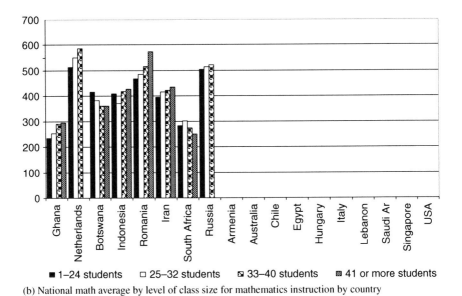

(b) National math average by level of class size for mathematics instruction by country

Fig. 9.4. The impact of class size for mathematics instruction on mathematics achievement

9.1.4 Class Size for Mathematics Instruction

Figure 9.4 (a) shows that class size was an inequity factor in eight countries out of the 18 countries in the sample. The percentage of variance of between-class mathematics achievement accounted for by this index ranged between 19% (Ghana) and 2% (Russian Federation). The bar graph 9.4(a) shows that six of those eight countries scored below TIMSS 2003 international average in TIMSS 2003 and five of those countries are developing countries.

There seems to be no consistent pattern in the way class size affects mathematics achievement. The direction of the impact of class size on mathematics achievement is controversial and most probably is context specific.

Class size is a factor that does not relate to any factor or attribute of the activity system of math education at the classroom/school level. In fact class size is related to two factors that are beyond the influence of the school: The education system as a whole and the socioeconomic level of the country.

9.2 Teacher Practices

Unlike the student practices, none of the teacher practices satisfied the conditions for inclusion in this chapter. TIMSS 2003 student and teacher background questionnaires included questions which asked students and teachers about their perceptions of the frequency of occurrence of some practices. Some of the practices were common to both questionnaires. Table 9.1 lists the six common practices and the number of countries in which the practice was an inequity factor. For each practice, the number of countries reflects the extent to which the practice was an inequity factor in math education across countries.

Table 9.1. Comparison of common student and teacher practices as inequity factors

Practice	Number of countries in which the practice was:	
	Teacher inequity factor	Student inequity factor
• Students explain answers in mathematics lessons	2	11
• Students work problems on their own in mathematics lessons	3	11
• Work together in small groups in mathematics lessons	5	8
• The teacher lecturing in mathematics lessons	4	4
• Relate what students are learning in mathematics to daily lives	3	2
• Students decide on their own procedures for solving complex problems in mathematics lessons	1	2

Table 9.1 shows that the extent to which student practices were inequity factors significantly exceeded that of teacher practices. The practice of 'having students explain their own answers in mathematics lessons' turned out to be a student inequity factor in 11 countries, compared to two countries for teachers. Similarly, the practice of enabling 'students to work problems on their own in mathematics lessons' turned out to be a student inequity factor in 11 countries, compared to three countries for teachers. It seems that students value their 'autonomy'.

9.3 Concluding Remarks

In this chapter four teacher indices were identified as inequity factors. On the other hand, no teacher practice was identified as an inequity factor. Table 9.2 lists the teacher indices which were inequity factors, the average strength of each, the number of countries in which the index was an inequity factor, and the interactions in the activity system that may account for the inequity in math achievement. Table 9.2 shows that the interactions of two or more of the following nodes (or their attributes) may account for the inequity in math achievement:

- Student: personal traits, socioeconomic, and cultural background
- Classroom community
- Math mediating artifacts
- Rules: School policies
- Education system
- Economic status of country

Table 9.2. Summary of teacher indices as inequity factors in the activity system

Inequity factor	Average strength	Number of countries	Interactions in the activity system that account for the inequity
▪ Index of Mathematics Teachers' Perception of School Climate	9.4	14	• School policies • Classroom community
▪ Index of Teachers' Reports on Teaching Mathematic Classes with Few or no Limitations on Instruction due to Student Factors	12.0	7	• Student and his/her attributes • Math mediating artifacts
▪ Index of Teachers' Emphasis on Mathematics Homework	3.2	6	• Math mediating artifacts
▪ Class Size for Mathematics Instruction	7.0	8	• Education system • Economic development of country

10

School-Related Inequity Factors

This chapter focuses on investigating the impact of school-related inequity factors based on the *TIMSS 2003 Principal Questionnaire* and TIMSS 2003 grade eight math assessment data. In this chapter, the school-related factors measure principals' perceptions of selected school and classroom practices. The dependent variable is the *The Average Plausible Score for the School (APSS)* in as much as they can be derived from *TIMSS 2003 Principal Questionnaire*. Since the original TIMSS school file did not include the mean math score of the students in the same teacher, a linkage program was developed to assign for each school principal the mean math score of students in that school. The (APSS) was computed to be the mean *Average of the Mathematics Plausible Score* (AMPS) for the students in the sample, who are in the same school (see Chapter 7). In this chapter, *A school-related inequity factor is defined to be a school-related factor that accounts for a significant percentage of the between-school variance (students in the same school)*.

For each of the 18 countries in the sample, a stepwise multiple regression was done with the school indices as predictors and (APSS) as a dependent variable. The stepwise multiple regression results are presented in a uniform pattern. An inequity factor is included in the discussion in this chapter, if it satisfies two conditions. First, the inequity factor should be significant, i.e. it should account for a significant (> 0) percentage of variance in APSS. Second, the inequity factor should be significant in at least six of the 18 countries in the sample. For each inequity factor that satisfies the two conditions, a figure consisting of a two-part bar graph is presented:

1. Sub-figure (a) represents the the inequity factor's strength (percentage of variance in the math achievement score accounted for by the inequity factor) for each country. It is used to identify the pattern of the inequity factor's strength across countries.
2. Sub-figure (b) represents the country's math average by inequity factor level for each country. It is used to identify the pattern of math mean differences associated with the levels of the inequity factor, across countries.

M. Jurdak, *Toward Equity in Quality in Mathematics Education*,
DOI 10.1007/978-1-4419-0558-1_10,
© Springer Science+Business Media, LLC 2009

The theoretical framework of the activity system at the school level will be used to interpret the significant inequity factors as interactions between the nodes of the system (Chapter 3). The rest of this chapter will be divided into sections, each presenting one school index.

10.1 Index of Principal Perception of School Climate

The index is computed from principals' responses regarding their characterization of the the following school climate factors: Teachers' job satisfaction, teachers' understanding of the school's curricular goals, teachers' degree of success in implementing the school's curriculum, teachers' expectations for student achievement, parental support for student achievement, parental involvement in school activities, students' regard for school property, and students' desire to do well in school.

Figure 10.1 (a) shows that this factor was an inequity factor in all countries in the sample except Hungary, Indonesia, Russian Federation, Saudi Arabia, and Italy. The percentage of variance of mathematics achievement accounted for by this index ranged between 59.8 (Lebanon) and 7.8% (Armenia). The bar graph 10.1 (a) shows that seven of the 18 countries are developing countries. It is remarkable that this index was an inequity factor in all but five countries in the sample and hence its impact cut across cultural, social, economic, and regional boundaries.

Figure 10.1 (b) shows that the more positive the principal's perception of school climate, the higher the mathematics achievement in each of the 13 countries in which this index was an inequity factor. The mean difference in mathematics achievement was most pronounced for the difference between the most and least positive perception of school climate (in favor of the former) and this difference was at least 50 points and reached a maximum of 135 points (equivalent to 1.35 standard deviations of TIMSS standardized score) in Botswana. The powerful impact of this index in 13 of the 17 countries in the sample indicates the extent to which the difference between high and low positive principal's high and low perception of school climate is associated with mathematics achievement.

School principal's perception of school climate is formed as a result of the principal's interaction with students, teachers, and the school community, especially the parents. Referring to the activity system at the school level (Figure 8.1), this index seems to relate to the interaction school of policies and culture, as well as, the home culture, as reflected in parental involvement and support for their children's. achievement.

Is school climate amenable to change by changing classroom practices or school policies? I believe it is. There is much that the school, especially its principal, can do to improve the its climate. Through its policies and practices, the school can directly influence many of the components of school climate. For example, the school can promote teachers' understanding of its curricular

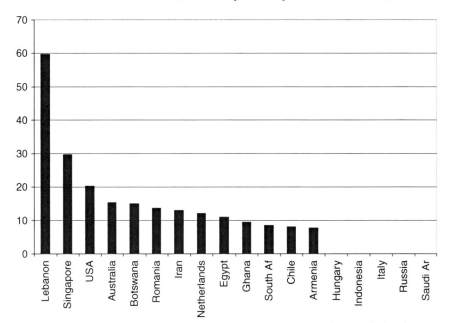

(a) Percentage of between- school variance in school math score accounted for by the index of principal perception of school climate, by country

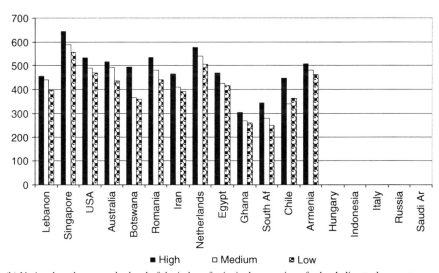

(b) National math average by level of the index of principal perception of school climate, by country

Fig. 10.1. The impact of principals' perception of school climate on math achievement

goals, support teachers in their efforts to n implement the school's curriculum, and to raise their expectations for student achievement. Also as an employer, the school can enhance teachers' job satisfaction. Moreover, the school can work with the students to improve their regard for school property and their desire to do well in school.

10.2 Index of Good School and Class Attendance

The index is computed from principals' responses to the frequency and severity of the following student behaviors: Arriving late at school, absenteeism, and skipping class. Figure 10.2 (a) shows that this factor was an inequity factor in nine countries. The percentage of variance of mathematics achievement accounted for by this index ranged between a remarkable 31.5 (Lebanon) and 1.9% (Singapore). The bar graph 10.2 (a) shows that three out of the nine countries are developing countries and six are developed countries. This factor had a moderate impact on school mathematics performance as judged by the number of countries, and it seems that its impact is relatively more in developed countries than in developing ones.

Figure 10.2 (b) shows that the higher the school and classroom attendance, the higher the school's mathematics achievement in each of the nine countries in which this index was an inequity factor. The mean difference in mathematics achievement was most pronounced for the difference between the 'high' and 'low' school and classroom attendance (in favor of the former) and this difference reached 74 points (equivalent to 0.74 standard deviations of TIMSS standardized score) in Iran.

Referring to the activity system of mathematics education at the school level (Figure 8.1), one can see that school attendance is mainly governed by the 'rules' in the activity system. In this case, the rules include school policies and the socioeconomic milieu. In this respect school policies lend themselves to change; however, it is difficult to manipulate the social component represented by the socioeconomic milieu of students and the perceptions of students and their parents of the 'value' of the education they are getting in school.

10.3 Concluding Remarks

In this chapter two of the three school-level indices were identified as inequity factors, namely, principal perception of school climate and Good School and Classroom Attendance. Both of the two indices are constituted by school policies and the socioeconomic milieu of students.

The other three school-level indices which did not meet the criteria to be inequity factors were: Index of Availability of School Resources for Mathematics Instruction, Number of Hours of School per Year, and Number of Weeks of

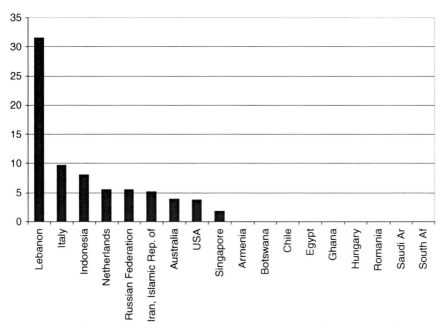

(a) Percentage of between-school variance in school math score accounted for by the index of good school and class attendance, by country

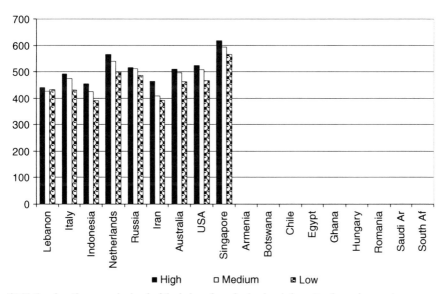

(b) National math average by level of the index of good school and class attendance, by country

Fig. 10.2. The impact of good school and class attendance on math achievement

School per Year. The availability of school resources for mathematics instruction is clearly related to the math mediating artifacts of the activity system.
One would have expected this index to have an impact on math achievement
in more than five countries on the basis that the availability of instructional
resources for math instruction enhances student math learning. The counter
argument is that it is not the availability of resources that is critical but rather
the way these resources are used and their appropriation by math teachers.

On the other hand, the the failure of number of hours (or weeks) per year
(both measures of the school year's length) to impact math achievement can
be rationalized on the basis of two considerations: First, it is the amount of
instructional time allotted to math that impacts math learning more than the
school year's length. Second, it is the quality of instruction that affects math
learning rather than than the time allotted for such instruction.

11

Global Inequity Factors

This chapter focuses on two objectives: First, the country-related inequity factors in math achievement are identified and examined. Second, the relationship between equity and quality of math education, at the country level, is explored. According to the definition in Chapter 7, a country-related inequity factor is one that accounts for a significant proportion of between-country variance in the country's TIMSS 2003 math score, as computed and published by TIMSS 2003. The country-related factors that will be considered in this chapter are the the country's educational and economic indicators.

The relationship between equity and quality at the country level, is explored through investigating the relationship between the country's math achievement and its inequity index, as measured by the between-school variance of total variance in math achievement. In this analysis, only the 18 countries in the sample are used.

The theoretical framework of the activity system at the global level will be used to interpret the inequity factors as interactions between the nodes of the system (Chapter 6). The 'subject' of this system is the country. For easy reference, the figure representing mathematics education as an activity system at the global level is reproduced, with factors and their attributes identified. The rest of this chapter will be divided into two sections, one dealing with country inequity factors and another with the relationship between equity and quality at the global level.

11.1 Country Indicators

11.1.1 Educational Indicators

The educational indicators were drawn from UNESCO Institute for Statistics mostly for the year 2005 (stats.uis.unesco.org). The selected educational indicators are:

1. School enrollment, primary (%net)

M. Jurdak, *Toward Equity in Quality in Mathematics Education*,
DOI 10.1007/978-1-4419-0558-1_11,
© Springer Science+Business Media, LLC 2009

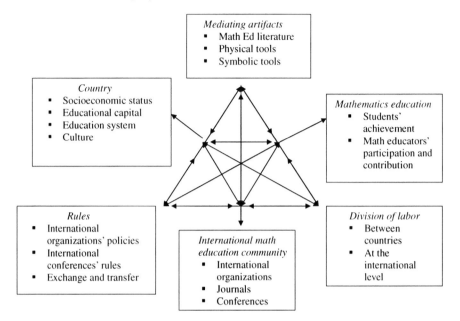

Fig. 11.1. Factors and their attributes in the activity system of mathematics education at the global level

2. School enrollment, primary (%gross)
3. school enrollment, secondary (%net)
4. School enrollment, secondary (%gross)
5. School enrollment, tertiary (%gross)
6. Children of primary school age who are out of school (%)
7. School life expectancy ISCED 1–6 years
8. Pupil teacher ratio (primary)
9. Expenditure on education as percentage of GDP
10. Expenditure on education as percentage of total government expenditure
11. Primary completion rate, total (percentage of relevant group)

11.1.2 Economic Educators

The economic indicators were taken from among the World Development Indicators on the World Bank web site (web.worldbank.org/wbsite/external/datastatistics). The selected economic indicators are:

1. Ratio of girls to boys in primary and secondary education
2. Adult literacy rate (percentage of people ages 15 and above)
3. Gross National Index(GNI)
4. Gross National Index per capita
5. Gross Domestic Product(GDP)

6. Poverty rate (percentage of population on less than 2 dollars per day)
7. Gross Domestic Product per capita
8. Gross Domestic Product growth rate(%)

11.2 Country Indicators and Mathematics achievement

In this section the 45 countries that had valid data in TIMSS 2003 were considered. A file for those countries was created and their respective economic and educational indicators were retrieved from UNESCO and World Bank home pages. The indicators that had significant correlations with the national mathematics score are listed in Table 11.1.

Table 11.1. Correlations of TIMSS national score to World Bank development indicators and UNESCO educational indicators

Economic indicators		Educational indicators	
Positive correlation			
• GDP per capita	+0.51	• Primary school net enrollment	+0.37
		• Secondary school net enrollment	+0.55
• GNI per capita	+0.43	• Tertiary enrollment	+0.61
		• School life expectancy	+0.37
		• Adult literacy	+0.63
Negative correlation			
• Poverty rate	−0.52	• % Out of school primary age children	−0.37
• Government expenditure on education	−0.37	• Primary pupil teacher ratio	−0.45

Three economic indicators had the highest impact on math achievement. The Gross Domestic Product (GDP) per capita and the Gross National Index (GNI) per capita correlated significantly and positively with the national mathematics achievement score. Poverty rate had a significant negative correlation with the national mathematics achievement score. The between-country variance in mathematics achievement accounted for by each of these three indicators was as follows:

1. GDP: 26%
2. GNI: 19%
3. Poverty rate: 27%

Three educational indicators had the highest impact on math achievement. These are the following, in descending order of impact on math achievement:

1. Adult literacy rate was positively correlated with the national math score and accounted for 40% of the between-country variance in it
2. Tertiary enrollment rate was positively correlated with the national math score and accounted for 37% of the between-country variance in it
3. Secondary school enrolment positively correlated with the national math score and accounted for 30% of the between-country variance in it

When the economic and educational indicators were entered in a stepwise multiple regression model, using the national math score as a dependent variable, tertiary enrollment rate was the only indicator that entered into the equation, accounting for 78% of the between-country variance in national math score. This indicates that, because of its partial correlation with the other indicators, the tertiary enrollment rate was the dominant indicator in the set of economic and educational indicators that were entered in the stepwise regression equation.

11.3 The Relationship Between Equity and Quality at the Country Level

11.3.1 Country Inequity Index

The *country math education inequity index* is defined as the percentage of between-school variance of total variance in the school math score in the country. The between-school variation is theoretically accounted for by variation in the aptitudes and attitudes of students attending different schools, and/or the quality of education provided by the schools. It is reasonable to assume that the aptitudes and attitudes of the students in the same country are more or less homogeneous across schools. Consequently, The between-school variance indicates the extent of variation among schools in mathematics achievement due to schools' educational quality. The larger the between-school variance in mathematics achievement in a country, the more is the inequity in educational provisions among schools in the country. The between-school variation was calculated for each country by using the variance component model taking the officially published national TIMSS 2003 mathematics score as a dependent variable and the school as a random variable.

Three levels of the country inequity index are defined as follows:

1. High inequity level: Country inequity index is > 60
2. Average inequity level: Country inequity index is between 60 and 40
3. Low inequity level: Country inequity index is < 40

The inequity index for each of the 18 countries in the sample is shown in Figure 11.2.

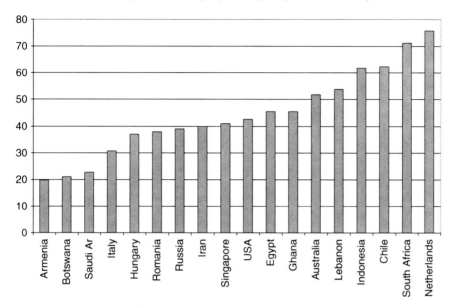

Fig. 11.2. Inequity index by country

11.3.2 Country Quality Index

In this chapter, the *country math quality index* is defined as the TIMSS 2003 national math score. Three levels were defined for the country quality index as follows:

1. High quality level: TIMSS 2003 country mathematics score is > 525
2. Average quality level: TIMSS 2003 country mathematics score is between 475 and 525
3. Low quality level: TIMSS 2003 country mathematics score is < 475

The quality index (TIMSS 2003 country mathematics score) by country is shown in Figure 11.3. By comparing Figures 11.2 and 11.3, one cannot discern a simple relationship between quality and inequity. For example, the highest three scoring countries, namely Singapore, Hungary, and the Netherlands have different inequity levels. The Netherlands has the highest inequity level, Singapore an average inequity level, and Hungary the lowest inequity level. On the other hand the lowest three scoring countries, namely Ghana, South Africa, and Saudi Arabia also differ in their inequity levels. South Africa had a very high inequity level, Ghana an average inequity level and Saudi Arabia a low inequity level.

11.3.3 Quality-Inequity Matrix

The 18 countries in the sample are mapped in a matrix whose two dimensions are quality and inequity. Nine countries were classified as low quality level in

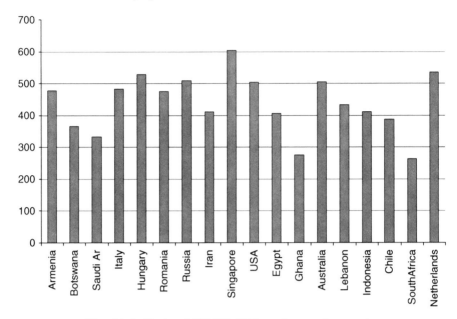

Fig. 11.3. National TIMSS 2003 math score by country

math education, six as average quality level, and three as high quality level. On the other hand, seven countries were classified as low inequity, seven as average inequity, and four as high inequity.

11.4 Optimal and Separate Modes of Development in Mathematics Education

The historical reasons for the emergence of a two-tiered system of math education at the global level were discussed in Chapter 6. The upper tier, which was called *the optimal mode of development* includes the developed countries which are integrated into the international mathematics education community. The lower tier, which was called *the separate mode of development* consists of the the marginalized countries which have yet to be included in the international activities of mathematics education.

A close examination of the quality-inequity matrix (Table 11.2) reveals that the nine countries having low quality index in math education (third row of Table 11.2) fit in the separate mode of development model. According to international comparative studies, these countries have low math performance, have little contribution to international research in mathematics education, and normally have humble participation in international mathematics education conferences such as the ICME's. In other words they are marginalized by

Table 11.2. Quality-inequity matrix for the 18 countries in the sample

		Quality Index		
		High	**Average**	**Low**
Equity Index	**High**	Hungary	Armenia Romania Russia Italy	Botswana Saudi Arabia
	Average	Singapore	United States Australia	Egypt Ghana Lebanon Iran
	Low	Netherlands		Chile Indonesia South Africa

the international mathematical education community and left to follow their own path in developing their mathematics education.

On the other hand, the other nine countries having average or high quality index fit the optimal mode of development model in math education. According to international comparative studies, these countries have high or average mathematics achievement performance, contribute significantly to international research in mathematics education, and assume leadership roles in international mathematics education organizations and conferences.

11.4.1 Contrasting the Developmental Profiles of Optimal and Separate Modes of Development

How do the developmental profiles of separate and optimal modes of development contrast in terms of developmental indicators? In Table 11.3, the 18 countries in the sample are classified according to their developmental mode in mathematics education (first column in the table), percentile rank of the country in terms of tertiary enrollment rate (column 3) and GNI per capita (column 4), and the region to which it belongs (column). A close examination of Table 11.3, supports the following assertions:

1. With the exception of Armenia, all the countries classified as fitting the optimal development mode, belong to three regions considered to be highly developed: North America, Western and Eastern Europe, East Asia and

the Pacific. On the other hand, with the exception of Indonesia, all the countries classified as following the separate development mode, belong to three regions considered to be developing: Arab states, Latin America, and Sub-saharan Africa.

Table 11.3. Percentile rank of tertiary enrollment rate and GNI per capita for each of the sample of countries classified by mode of development and region

Development mode	Country	Tertiary enrollment rate	GNI per capita	Region
Optimal development	-Armenia	20	20	-Central Asia
	-Australia	80	90	-East Asia and the Pacific
	-Hungary	70	70	-Central and Eastern Europe
	-Italy	70	90	-North America and Western Europe
	-Netherlands	70	100	-North America and Western Europe
	-Romania	60	40	-Central and Eastern Europe
	-Russian Federation	80	40	-Central and Eastern Europe
	-Singapore	–	80	-East Asia and the Pacific
	-United States	100	100	-North America and Western Europe
Separate development	-Botswana	10	50	-Sub-Saharan Africa
	-Chile	60	50	-Latin America and the Carribean
	-Egypt	40	10	-Arab States
	-Ghana	10	10	-Sub-Saharan Africa
	-Indonesia	20	10	-East Asia and the Pacific
	-Iran, Islamic Rep.of	20	10	-South and West Asia
	-Lebanon	60	50	-Arab States
	-Saudi Arabia	20	70	-Arab States
	-South Africa	10	50	-Sub-Saharan Africa

2. With regard to GNI per capita, Six of the nine optimal development countries are in the upper 30% of the countries in the sample in terms of GNI per capita. For the nine separate development countries, eight of them are in the lower 50% of the countries in the sample, four of which are in the lowest 10%.
3. With regard to tertiary enrollment ratio, seven of the nine optimal development countries are in the upper 30% of the countries in the sample; whereas, six of the nine separate development countries are in the lowest 20%.
4. More or less, the classification of countries along the line of mode of development in math education approximates the well-known north-south division in terms of geography, economy, and education.

In summary a country classified as fitting in the separate mode of development of mathematics education is likely to be relatively poor, low in the spread and level of education among its population, and belongs to a socioeconomically developing region. On the other hand, a country classified as following the optimal mode of development of mathematics education is likely to be relatively rich, high in the spread and level of education among its population, and is part of a developed region.

11.5 Concluding remarks

There seems to be a divide between developing and developed countries in mathematics education and the factors that contribute to that divide seem to be out of the reach of math educators and even national governments. Factors such as poverty or wealth of a country or the spread and level of education of its population cannot be changed immediately by national policies.

Referring to the activity system at the global level (Figure 11.1), one can account for the inequity in math education between countries in terms of interaction between the following four factors and their attributes in the activity system at the global level as follows:

1. Country: Socioeconomic status and educational capital
2. International math community: Participation in international math education organizations and in production of math education knowledge
3. Rules: Policies that govern international organizations and conferences
4. Division of labor: Power relationships among countries
5. Math mediating artifacts: English as the international language in math education and access to international math education literature

12

Epilogue

This chapter is both an overview of and a reflection on the findings in the previous chapters. Specifically, the chapter has four parts. First, it presents some generalizations based on both the theoretical analysis and the critical review of equity-related literature that were presented in Part I of the book. Second, it revisits the multilevel math education activity system from a cross-layer perspective. Third, it presents an overview of the analysis of TIMSS data in Part II. Fourth, it presents my personal reflection on how to proceed towards equity in quality in math education.

12.1 Some Generalizations

In Part I of the book the theoretical framework of the activity system was introduced and then used as an analytic tool to synthesize and discuss equity-related literature in math education. The following assertions are tenable within the assumptions and the findings of Part I.

Inequities result from interactions of the activity system factors: The activity system factors and their attributes are by themselves neutral to equity or inequity; it is the interaction of these factors and their attributes that may make them inequitable.

Inequities are amenable to change by changing policies or practices: The definition of an inequity factor as being the result of interaction among activity system factors and their attributes implies that inequity factors are amenable to change, in principle, by changing policies or practices that govern the interaction of the relevant factors and their attributes. In other words, inequities are not innate in individuals and groups but come as a result of their interactions in achieving the objects of purposeful human activities.

Inequities in the activity system are interdependent: The factors of the activity system are related horizontally and longitudinally. Horizontally, for

M. Jurdak, *Toward Equity in Quality in Mathematics Education*,
DOI 10.1007/978-1-4419-0558-1_12,
© Springer Science+Business Media, LLC 2009

each level of the activity system (school, national, and global), inequities are due to the interactions among the factors in the system. Longitudinally, the elements of a system at one level are related to the elements of the system at another level by a hierarchical relation of inclusion. For example, gender is a factor under 'student' in the school system and as such it interacts with other factors in the mathematics education activity system at the school level to produce inequities. On the other hand, if gender as an inequity factor becomes prevalent in many schools, it may become an inequity factor among schools in the mathematics education system at the country level.

12.2 A Cross-Layer Perspective of the Math Education Activity System

The math education activity system is a complex multi-layer system of at least three layers: School, country, and world. In Chapters 4, 5, and 6 the three layers were examined respectively as horizontal isolated systems. In this section, the cross-layer vertical relation between the three systems is explored. Figure 12.1 is a visual representation of the three layers horizontally and vertically.

The three layers are linked by hierarchical and nested relationships. The nested relationship is reflected in two aspects. On the one hand, each system becomes the 'subject' in the higher system which immediately follows. For example, the school system is the 'subject' in the country and the country system is the 'subject' in the global system. On the other hand, each attribute of a factor in one system is a part of the corresponding part of the next higher system. For example, the socioeconomic background of the student in the school system contributes to the determination of the socioeconomic constituency of the school in the country system. The nested relationship is not only that of inclusion but also a hierarchical power relationship. This suggests that societal relationships of a given system are present in each subsystem and consequently, relationships of power and influence carry over to the subjects in the subsystems and eventually affect the student activity system at the classroom level. As a result of the nested hierarchical relationship across the three layers, the inequity factors carry over from one system to the other.

The table in Figure 12.2, lists the attributes of each of 'subject', 'community', 'math mediating artifacts', and 'division of labor' at the level of each of school, country, and global systems as identified in Chapters 4, 5, an 6 respectively. The two factors of 'rules' and 'mathematics learning' are practically the same for all three layers and hence are not included in Figure 12.2. The attributes were then compared across the three layers to identify the 'common attributes'. For example, in the 'subject' column of Figure 12.2, comparison revealed that the attributes of 'socioeconomic level' and 'culture' are common to the 'subject' factor in each of school, country, and global systems.

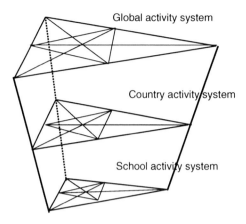

Fig. 12.1. A visual representation of the multi-layer structure of the mathematics education activity system

Subject	Community	Mediating Artifacts	Division of Labor
School Level			
Student • Personal traits (gender, ethnicity, native language...) • Socio-economic background • Cultural background	*Classroom community* • Constituency • Organization • Interactions	• Physical tools • Symbolic tools	• Between students • Between student and teachers
National Level			
School • Constituency • Resources • Climate	*Educational system community* • Differentiation • Decentralization	• Physical tools • Symbolic tools • Mandated or recommended artifacts	• Between schools • Between school and state • Privatization
Global Level			
Country • Socioeconomic status • Educational capital • Education system • Culture	*International math education community* • International organizations • Journals • Conferences	• Physical tools • Symbolic tools • Mandated or recommended artifacts	• Between countries • Within the international community

Fig. 12.2. A longitudinal view of the inequity factors across school, national, and global activity systems

This cross-layer comparison was done for the remaining factors. The common attributes that were identified for each factor are:

1. *Subject*
   - Socioeconomic status
   - Culture
2. *Community*
   - Structure
   - Organization
3. *Mediating artifacts*
   - Material artifacts for mathematics instruction and learning
   - Natural and mathematical languages
4. *Mathematics learning*
   - Achievement
   - Participation
5. *Division of labor*
   - Between the 'subject' and community members
   - Within the community
6. *Rules*
   - Institutional policies
   - Sociocultural norms

12.3 Interpretation of TIMSS 2003 Data Analysis Through the Activity System Lens

The table in Figure 12.3 is an overview of the findings from TIMSS analysis. It lists the significant inequity factors that relate to student (Chapter 8), teacher/classroom (Chapter 9), school (Chapter 10), and the global context (Chapter 11). The table also lists the interactions of the activity system that account for each of those inequity factors.

It is remarkable that the activity system framework was capable of accounting for all significant inequity factors at all levels in terms of interactions of its factors and their attributes. This implies that the activity system framework has the capability of being, not only an analytic framework to synthesize and analyze research studies, but also as an interpretative framework for inequity in math education.

12.4 System-Wise Transformation to Achieve Equity In Quality

Moving towards equity in quality is not likely to be achieved without a system-wise transformation i.e, a transformed relationship among the elements of the

Inequity factor	Interactions in the activity system that account for the inequity
Student	
▪ Index of Self-Confidence in Learning Mathematics	● Student cultural background ● Math mediating artifacts
▪ Index of Student Educational Aspirations Relative to Parents Educational Level	● Classroom community ● Student socioeconomic background
▪ Index of Parent Highest Education Level	● Student ● Classroom community
▪ Index of Student Perception of Being Safe in School	● Rules ● Classroom community
▪ Use of computer	● Math mediating artifacts ● Student socioeconomic background
Teacher/Classroom	
▪ Index of Mathematics Teachers' Perception of School Climate	● School policies ● Classroom community
▪ Index of Teachers' Reports on Teaching Mathematic Classes with Few or no Limitations on Instruction due to Student Factors	● Student and its attributes ● Math mediating artifacts
▪ Index of Teachers' Emphasis on Mathematics Homework	● Math mediating artifacts
▪ Class Size for Mathematics Instruction	● Education system ● Economic development of country
School	
▪ Index of Principal Perception of School Climate	▪ School policies ▪ The socioeconomic milieu of students
▪ Index of Good School and Class Attendance	▪ School policies ▪ The socioeconomic milieu of students
Country	
▪ Participation in international math education organizations and in production of math education knowledge	▪ Country's SES and educational capital ▪ International math community ▪ International policies ▪ Division of labor: Power relationships ▪ Math mediating artifacts: English language and access to literature

Fig. 12.3. Interpretation of TIMSS-based inequity factors through the activity system lens

system. The hierarchical and nested structure of the math education activity system raises a question about where to start this transformation. Can the math teacher move towards equity in quality or does she or he need to wait until the school system starts to be transformed in that direction? Similarly, can the school move towards equity in quality or does it need to wait until the national system starts to move in that direction? I believe the answer to both questions is negative so long as the constraints and limitations of the hierarchical nested structure of the activity system are recognized.

The math teacher, for example, can systematically address some of the inequity issues in the classroom, such as building students' self-concepts, and asking students to explain their answers. Although this effort is within the and/or activity domain of the teacher, it is likely to be constrained by school policies parental and school expectations regarding meeting achievement standards. Similarly, the school can start a systematic process towards addressing some of the inequities in it, such as improving the school climate. Again, those efforts may be constrained by the policies of the educational system to which the school belongs and which govern relations of teachers, students, and school administration.

12.4.1 Transformation in the Activity System

According to Engeström (1999), the development or *transformation* of an activity system takes place through an *expansive cycle* which refers to a qualitative change that results in a new activity system to replace the preceding one. These expansive cycles are triggered by 'formation and resolution of internal contradictions' p. 33. These contradictions can be within a factor (node) of the system, between different nodes in the system, or between different systems.

According to Engeström (1999), the expansive cycle of an activity system follows a certain pattern:

1. 'An almost exclusive emphasis on internalization, on socializing and training the novices to become competent members of the activity system as it is routinely carried out' p. 33. 'Internalization is the transition in which external processes with external, material objects are transformed into processes that take place at the mental level, the level of consciousness' (Zinchencho & Gordon, 1981, p. 74)
2. Participants in the activity engage in *externalization*-a process of inventing ways and artifacts as they implement their learning in different contexts. Externalization 'occurs first in the form of discrete individual innovations' p. 33
3. As a result of disruptions and contradictions during practice, 'internalization increasingly takes the form of critical self-reflection and externalization, a search for solutions increases' p. 34
4. A new model of the individual activity emerges as externalization reaches its peak
5. The successful orchestration of the collective emerging of individual activities will be an expansive cycle to eventually stabilize as a new activity system

12.5 System-Wise Transformation: The Case of Lebanon

In this section I present an example of how a national system could be transformed to achieve equity in quality in math education. The example is that of Lebanon, my home country. In this example, Lebanon is used as a real context to demonstrate a suggested strategy for a system-wise transformation towards equity in quality. In giving this example I make the following assumptions:

1. Mathematics education is a nested hierarchical multilayered activity system.
2. The activity system of mathematics education is unique in its structure, content, and history. It is also assumed that the subsidiary activity systems are also unique and diverse in their history and expectations.
3. The inequities in the activity system and its subsidiaries constitute potential sources of imbalances and contradictions in the system and these are likely to activate a process towards an expansive cycle in the system to achieve equity i.e. stability in the system.
4. There should be a political will at the policy-making level to achieve equity in quality.

12.5.1 The Context

Lebanon is a small country of about four million people. Historically it was a crossroad of many civilizations and now stands as a bridge between the West and the Arab World. Lebanese society is multicultural and trilingual (Arabic, English, French). Lebanon became an independent state in 1943.

Because of historical reasons, the Lebanese education system has special features. First, the public education system caters to only 40% of pre-university students, while private schools, many of which were established by religious missionaries and organizations, cater to the remaining 60% of the students. Public schools accommodate students coming from mostly low socioeconomic classes, while private schools accommodate students coming from middle and high socioeconomic classes. Second, math and science are taught in either English or French and not in the native language of Arabic.

12.5.2 The Inequity

Lebanon participated in TIMSS for the first time in 2003. Though it ranked first among the eight Arab countries that participated in grade eight TIMSS 2003, it scored 433 which is 67 points below the international TIMSS 2003 average. Subsequent analysis revealed that private schools had a significantly higher mean TIMSS score than public schools.

A study conducted by The Lebanese Center for Educational Research and Development (CERD) examined the trends in student math scores of the national government examination (Brevet), given at the end of grade 9. On the average, results indicate that private schools did better than public schools. This difference was accounted for by student proficiency in the foreign language in which math was taught.

In Chapter 11 of this book, the analysis of TIMSS 2003 data indicated that, in Lebanon, 45% of of variance in TIMSS math score was accounted for by variation between schools. This was rather on the high side compared to other countries. It also indicates that the type of school accounts significantly for math achievement differences.

Research evidence, as well as public perception points to the existence of an inequity in math achievement between private and public schools. It is clear that this inequity is due to complex interactions of many factors in the national activity system. Among other things, these factors include the school's constituency, resources and climate; the math learning artifacts, especially language of instruction; decentralization of the education system and national educational policies.

12.5.3 The Conflict

The inequity in math education between private and public schools contradicts Lebanon's adopted goal of education for all. Lebanon formally adopted the goals of Education For All (EFA) as reflected in the Dakar Framework for Action (UNESCO, 2000). One of the Dakar Framework's goals is 'improving all aspects of the quality of education and ensuring excellence of all so that recognized and measurable learning outcomes are achieved by all, especially in literacy, numeracy and essential life skills.' It is clear that there is a contradiction between inequity in math achievement and the declared goals of EFA. To resolve this conflict the educational authority needs to develop a strategic plan.

12.5.4 A Suggested Strategy

Adopting of a strategic equity goal: In the case of Lebanon, the educational authority should reaffirm its commitment to providing equity in the quality of math education. A strategic goal is to be formulated to encompass the depth and extent of the commitment of the 'actors' in the system toward equity and quality. It also should incorporate the envisioned transformed activity system. The following is a an example of a widely-encompassing formulation of an equity in quality strategic goal that could be formulated in this case.

> 'Equal access to high quality mathematics education for all students, schools, and regions in the country'

All indicators affirm that public school math achievement was lower than that of private schools. Hence, the objective is to improve the quality of math education in public schools.

Identifying the possible sources of inequity in math in public schools: This process requires the identification of system factors whose interactions could be possible sources of the underachievement in public schools. These factors should lend themselves to change by changing policies or practices. In this case, possible factors are: School resources and climate; math learning artifacts, especially language of instruction and teachers' pedagogical content knowledge; and school autonomy. The identification of such factors may require more research to determine the strength of the impact of these factors on inequity in achievement.

Developing a comprehensive action plan: The action plan is supposed to be aligned with the strategic equity goal. Probably in this case, the action plan would be at three levels:

- National educational authority: To develop and adopt the needed policies such as increasing school autonomy, foreign language instruction in public schools, as well as providing the needed financial and material resources for public schools
- Public school: To translate the adopted policies into school policies and practices that are meaningful and suitable within the school context. These include things like school climate and resources for math instruction
- Math teacher: To use the school resources and the acquired equity-related pedagogical knowledge to promote equity in math classroom practices

Preparing professional development programs: The professional development programs should focus on how to improve the quality of math education of public schools students by catering for their special needs. Below are some examples of topics that may be included in the professional development programs of public school principals and math teachers.

- Math teacher: Teaching math in a foreign language, providing for special needs in math instruction, preparing remedial and enrichment math instructional and learning materials.
- Principal: Assuming the role of an instructional leader, ways to improve school climate, using the community resources to enhance math learning at school

Delivering the professional development to principals and teachers: School principals and math teachers will start to learn about the actions and practices that supposedly serve the strategic goal of equity in quality. At this stage, the principals and teachers internalize these actions and practices as knowledge at the cognitive level.

Undertaking reflective practice by school principals and math teachers: School principals start to implement the new policies and math teachers start to use the newly-acquired pedagogical content knowledge in their classroom teaching. During this phase, principals and teachers attempt to optimize their new knowledge to their actual work contexts. In doing so, they engage in a process of self-reflection on their own practices.

Transformation at the level of individual schools and teachers: The process of reflective practice will eventually lead the individual principals and math teachers to adapt and eventually adopt the equity practices as they apply to their own specific work contexts. This indicates that the process of transformation has occurred at the individual level.

Towards equity in quality in math education in public schools: Each public school makes sure that the practices of math teachers are aligned with the equity strategic goal. The alignment of the practices of all public schools with the equity strategic goal is an indicator of the transformation of the public education system towards more equitable math education.

The road to equity in quality is long and difficult and it requires the transformation of individuals as well as of the system itself. It is the orchestration of the individual and system-wise transformations that makes the realization of the strategic goal of equity in quality difficult but hopeful. It is difficult because first, the system itself has to be transformed in order to achieve equity in quality, and second, the transformation of the system is constrained by the nested hierarchical structure of the activity system. On the other hand, it is hopeful because the role of the individual actor is essential for the transformation of the system. The need to orchestrate individual and collective activities is what makes the change possible and sustainable.

References

Chapter 1

Bourdieu, P., Passcron, J. C., & de Saint Martin. (1994). In Bourdieu, P., Passcron, J. C., & de Saint Martin (Eds.), *Academic discourse: Linguistic misunderstanding and professional power* (pp. 35–79). Stanford: Stanford University Press.

Engeström, Y. (1987). *Learning by expanding: An activity theoretical approach to developmental research.* Helsinki: Orienta-Konsultit Oy.

Griffiths, V. (1953). *An experiment in education.* London: Longmans.

Leont'ev, A. N. (1981).The problem of activity in psychology. In Wertsch (Ed.), *The concept of activity in Soviet psychology* (pp. 37–71). New York: M. E. Sharpe, Armonk.

Jurdak, M. E. (1973). *The effects of emphasising mathematics structural properties in teaching and of reflective intelligence on four selected criteria.* Madison, WI: The Wisconsin R & Development Center for Cognitive Learning.

Jurdak, M. E. (1977). Structural and linguistics variables in selected inference patterns for bilinguals in grades six to ten. *Educational Studies in Mathematics, 8,* 225–238.

Jurdak, M. E., & Jacobsen, E. (1981). The evolution of mathematics curricula in the Arab States. In R. Morris (Ed.), *Studies in mathematics education: Vol. 2* (pp. 133–147). Paris: UNESCO.

Jurdak, M. E., & Mutlak, I. (1982). The facilitating effect of structured games in mathematics. *International Journal of Mathematics Education in Science and Technology, 13,* 335–340.

Jurdak, M. E. (1985). The role of sequence and context in structurally-related problems. *International Journal of Mathematical Education in Science and Technology, 16,* 515–524.

Jurdak, M. E. (1989). Religion and language as culture carriers and barriers in mathematics education. In C. Kietel (Ed.), *Mathematics, Education and Society (Science and Technology Education, Document Series No. 35),* pp. 12–14, Paris: UNESCO.

Jurdak, M. E. (1994). Mathematics education in the global village. In D. Robitaille, D. Wheeler, & C. Kieran (Eds.), *Selected lectures from the 7th International Congress on Mathematical Education* (pp. 199–210). Quebec: Laval University.

Jurdak, M., & Shahin, I. (1999). An ethnographic study of the computational strategies of a group of young street vendors in Beirut. *Educational Studies in Mathematics, 40*, 155–172.

Jurdak, M. (2001). Contrasting problem- solving in school and workplace. In Pehkonen, E. (Ed.), *Problem solving around the world* (pp. 97–102). Turku: University of Turku.

Jurdak, M., & Shahin, I. (2001). Problem solving activity in the workplace and the school: The case of constructing solids. *Educational Studies in Mathematics, 47*, 297–315.

Jurdak, M. (2006a). Contrasting perspectives and performance of high school students on problem solving in real world, situated, and school contexts. *Educational Studies in Mathematics, 63*, 283–301.

Jurdak, M. (2006b). *Impact of student, teacher, school factors on achievement in mathematics and science based on TIMSS 2003 Arab Countries Data.* Beirut: UNESCO Regional Office in Beirut (limited distribution)

Chapter 2

Begle, E. (1970). Introduction. In E. Begle (Ed.), *Mathematics education: The sixty-ninth yearbook of the National Society for the Study of Education (NSSE)* (pp. 1–4). Chicago, IL: NSSE.

Board on Mathematical Sciences and Mathematical Sciences Education Board. (1989). *Everybody counts: A report to the nation on the future of mathematics education.* Washington, DC: National Research Council

Bruner, J. (1960). *The process of education.* Cambridge: Harvard University Press. Chicago, IL: NSSE.

Committee of Inquiry into the Teaching of Mathematics in Schools. (1982). *The cockcroftrreport: Mathematics counts.* http://www.dg.dial.pipex.com/documents/docs1/cockcroft.shtml

Delores, J. et al. (1996). *Learning: The treasure within, report of the International Commission on Education for the twenty-first century.* http://www.unesco.org/delors/delors_e.pdf

Faure, E. et al. (1972). *Learning to be: The world of education of today and tomorrow. Report by the International Commission on the Development of Education.* Paris: Unesco.

Fulvia Furinghetti and Livia Giacardi. *History of ICMI.* http://www.icmihistory.unito.it/congress.php

Gates, P. (2006). The place of equity and social justice in the history of PME. In A. Guitierres & P. Boero (Eds.), *Handbook of research on the psychology of mathematics education: Past, present, and future* (pp. 367–402). Rotterdam: Sense Publishers.

Hanna, G. (Ed.). (1996). *Towards gender equity in mathematics education – ICMI study.* Boston, MA: Kluwer

Leung, K. et al. (2006). *Mathematics education in different cultural traditions – A comparative study of East Asia and the west, ICMI study.* Boston, MA: Springer

Morris, R. (1981). *Studies in mathematics education, Volume 2.* Paris: UNESCO.

National Council of Teachers of Mathematics (NCTM). (2000). *Principles and standards for school mathematics.* http://standardstrial.nctm.org/document/chapter2/index.htm

National Society for the Study of Education (NSSE). (1951). *The teaching of arithmetic.* Chicago, IL:NSSE.

National Society for the Study of Education. (NSSE). (1970). *Mathematics education: The Sixty-ninth Yearbook of the National Society for the Study of Education (NSSE).* Chicago, IL: NSSE.

Niss, M. (1996). Goals of mathematics teaching. In A.J. Bishop et al. (Eds), *International handbook of mathematics education* (pp. 11–47). Boston, MA: Kluwer.

Qualifications and Curriculum Authority (QCA). (1999). *National curriculum: Values, aims and purposes key stages 1 and 2.* http://curriculum.qca.org.uk/key-stages-1-and-2/Values-aims-and-purposes/index.aspx

Qualifications and Curriculum Authority (QCA). (2007). *National curriculum: Values, aims and purposes key stages 3 and 4.* http://curriculum.qca.org.uk/key-stages-3-and-4/aims/index.aspx

UNESCO. (1969). *School mathematics in the Arab countries, UNESCO mathematics project for the Arab States* (SC/WS/201). Paris: UNESCO.

UNESCO. (1966). *UNESCO pilot project for the Improvement of mathematics teaching in the Arab States* (WS/1266/101/AVS/DST). Paris: UNESCO.

UNESCO. (1990). *World Conference on Education for All.* Jomtien, Thailand, 5–9 March, 1990.http://www.unesco.org/education/efa/ed_for_all/background/jomtien_declaration.shtml

UNESCO. (2000). *The Dakar framework for action: Education for all – meeting our collective commitments.* World Education Forum, Dakar, Senegal, 26–28 April. http://www.unesco.org/education/efa/ed_for_all/dakfram_eng.shtml

UNESCO. (2004). *Education for all: The quality imperative.* Paris: UNESCO.

United Nations. (1948). *Universal Declaration of Human Rights, Article 26.* http://www.un.org/Overview/rights.html

United Nations. (1966a). *International Covenant on Civil and Political Rights* (ICCPR). http://www.hrweb.org/legal/cpr.html

United Nations. (1966b). *International Covenant on Economic, Social and Cultural Rights* (ICESCR). http://www.unhchr.ch/html/menu3/b/a_cescr.htm

United Nations. (2000). *Millennium Declaration.* http://www.un.org/millennium-goals/

Wilder R. (1970). Historical background of innovations in mathematics curricula. In E. Begle (Ed.), *Mathematics education: The Sixty-ninth Yearbook of the National Society for the Study of Education (NSSE),* 7–22. Chicago, IL: NSSE.

Chapter 3

Atweh, B., Forgas, H., & Nebres, B. (Eds.). (2001). *Socio-cultural research on mathematics education-An international perspective.* London: Lawrence Erlbaum Associates Publishers.

Berne, R., & L. Stiefel. (1984). *The measurement of equity in school finance: Conceptual, methodological, and empirical dimensions.* Baltimore, MD: The Johns Hopkins University Press.

Burton, L. (Ed.). (2003). *Which way social justice in mathematics education?* Westport: Praeger Publishers.

Christiansen, I. (2007). Some tensions in mathematics education for democracy. *The Montana Mathematics Enthusiast*, http://www.montanamath.org/TMME Monograph 1, 49–62.

Engeström, Y. (1987). *Learning by expanding: An activity theoretical approach to developmental research.* Helsinki: Orienta-Konsultit Oy.

Engeström,Y. (1999). Activity theory and individual and social transformation. In Y. Engeström, R. Miettinen, & R.-L. Punamaki (Eds.), *Perspctives on activity theory* (pp. 19–38), Cambridge: Cambridge University Press.

Hanushek, E., & Luque, J. (2003). Efficiency and equity in schools around the world. *Economics Education Review, 22*, 481–502.

Jurdak, M., & Shahin, I. (1999). An ethnographic study of the computational strategies of a group of young street vendors in Beirut. *Educational Studies in Mathematics Education, 40*, 155–172.

Jurdak, M. (2006). *Impact of student, teacher, school factors on achievement in mathematics and science based on TIMSS 2003 Arab Countries Data.* Beirut: UNESCO Regional Office in Beirut (130 pages), (limited distribution).

Leont'ev, A. N. (1981). The problem of activity in psychology. In Wertsch (Ed.), *The concept of activity in Soviet psychology* (pp. 37–71). New York: M. E. Sharpe, Armonk.

Noyes, A. (2007). Mathematical marginalisation and meritocracy: Inequity in an English classroom. *The Montana Mathematics Enthusiast*, Monograph 1, 35–48 http://www.montanamath.org/TMME

Paavola, S., Lipponen, L., & Hakkarainen, K. (2004). Models of innovative knowledge communities and three metaphors of learning. *Review of Educational Research, 74*, 557–576.

PISA. (2005). *School factors related to quality and equity: Results from PISA 2000.* Paris: OECD Publishing.

Secada,W., Fennema, E., & Byrd-Adajian, L. (1995). *New directions for equity in mathematics education.* New York: Cambridge University Press.

Sfard, A. (1998). On two metaphors of learning and the dangers of choosing one. *Educational Researcher, 27*, 4–13

Sriraman, B. (2007). 0n the origins of social justice: Darwin, Freire, Marx and Vivekananda. *The Montana Mathematics Enthusiast*, Monograph 1, 1–6 http://www.montanamath.org/TMME

UNESCO. (2005). *Education for all-the quality imperative, summary.* Paris: UNESCO

Valero, P., & Zeverbergen, R.(Eds.). (2004). *Researching the socio-political dimensions of mathematics education: Issues of power in theory and methodology.* Dordrecht: Kluwer.

Zinchenko V. P., & Gordon V. M. (1981). Methodological problems in analyzing activity, In Wertsch (Ed.), *The concept of activity in Soviet psychology* (pp. 37–71). NY: M.E. Sharpe, Armonk.

Chapter 4

Adler, J. (2001). Resourcing practice and equity: A dual challenge for mathematics education. In B. Atweh, H. Forgasz, & B. Nebres (Eds.), *Sociocultural research on mathematics education: An international Perspective* (pp. 185–200). Mahwah, NJ: Lawrence Erlbaum Associates, Publishers.

Baker, D., & Street, B. (2000). Math as social explanation for 'underachievement' in numeracy. In T. Nakahara & M. Koyama (Eds.), *Proceedings of the 24th PME International Conference, 2,* 49–56.

Bartholomew, H. (2004). Equity and empowerment in mathematics: Some tensions from the secondary classroom. In I. Putt et al. (Eds.), *Proceedings of MERGA 27: Mathematics education for the third millennium, 1,* 71–78.

Barwell, R. (2001). Investigating mathematical interactions in a multilingual primary school: Finding a way of working. In M. van den Heuvel-Panhuizen (Ed.), *Proceedings of the 25th PME International Conference, 2,* 97–104.

Boaler, J. (1997). Setting, social class, and the survival of the quickest. *British Educational Research Journal, 23,* 575–595.

Boaler, J. (2002). Learning from teaching: Exploring the relationship between reform curriculum and equity. *Journal for Research in Mathematics Education, 33,* 239–258.

Bourdieu, P., Passcron, J. C., & de Saint Martin. (1994). In Bourdieu, P., Passcron, J. C., & de Saint Martin (Eds.), *Academic discourse: Linguistic misunderstanding and professional power* (pp. 35–79). Stanford: Standford University Press.

Burris, C., Heubert, J., & Levin, H. (2006). Accelerating mathematics achievement using heterogeneous grouping. *American Educational Research Journal, 43,* 105–136.

Cobb, P., & Hodge, L., (2002). A relational perspective on issues of cultural diversity and equity as they play out in the mathematics classroom. *Mathematical. Thinking and Learning, 4,* 249–284.

D'Ambrosio, U. (1985). Ethnomathematics and its place in the history of pedagogy of mathematics. *For the Learning of Mathematics, 5,* 44–48.

Forgasz, H. (2003). Equity,and beliefs about the efficacy of computers for mathematics learning. In N. A. Pateman, B. J. Dougherty, & J. T. Zilliox (Eds.), *Proceedings of the 27th PME International Conference, 2,* 381–388.

Forgasz, H. (2004). Equity and computers for mathematics learning: access and attitudes. In M. J. Hoines & A. B. Fuglestad (Eds.), *Proceedings of the 28th PME International Conference, 2,* 399–406.

Forgasz, H. (2006). Teachers, equity, and computers for secondary mathematics learning. *Journal of Mathematics Teacher Education, 9,* 437–469.

Frempong, G. (2005). Exploring excellence and equity within Canadian mathematics classrooms. In Chick, L. & Vincent, L. (Eds.), *Proceedings of the 29th PME International Conference, 2,* 237–244.

Gerdes, P. (1988). On culture, geometrical thinking and mathematics education. *Educational Studies in Mathematics Education, 19, 137–162.*

Gorgorio, N., & Planas, N. (2001). Teaching mathematics in multilingual classrooms. *Educational Studies in Mathematics, 47,* 7–33.

Gutierrez, R. (2008). A 'gap-gazing' fetish in mathematics education? Problematizing research on the achievement gap. *Journal for Research in Mathematics Education, 34,* 37–73.

Gutstein, E. (2003). Teaching and learning mathematics for social justice. *Journal for Research in Mathematics Education, 39,* 357–364.

Gutstein, E. (2007). Multiple language use and mathematics: Politicizing the discussion. *Educational Studies in Mathematics, 64,* 243–246.

Jurdak, M., & Shahin, I. (1999). An ethnographic study of the computational strategies of a group of young street vendors in Beirut. *Educational Studies in Mathematics, 40,* 155–172.

Jurdak, M. E. (1989). Religion and language as culture carriers and barriers in mathematics education. In C. Kietel (Ed.), *Mathematics, education and society (Science and Technology Education, Document Series No. 35)* (pp. 12–14). Paris: UNESCO.

Kahn, M. (2005). A class act-mathematics as a filter of equity in South Africa. *Perspectives in Education, 23,* 139–148.

Khisty, L., & Chval, K. (2002). Pedagogic discourse and equity in mathematics: When teachers talk matters. *Mathematics Education Research Journal, 14,* 154–168.

Kutscher, B., & Linchevski, L. (2000). Moving between mixed-ability and same-ability settings: Impact upon learners. In T. Nakahara & M. Koyama (Eds.), *Proceedings of the 24th PME International Conference, 3,* 199–206.

Leder, G. (2004). Mathematics, gender, and equity issues-another perspective. In B. Clarke et al. (Eds.), *International overboard! The complexities perspectives on learning and teaching mathematics* (pp. 253–266). Goteborg: Goteborg University.

Lerman, S. (2003). Developing theories of mathematics education research: The PME story. *Educational Studies in Mathematics, 51,* 23–40.

Ma, X. (2008). Gender differences in mathematics achievement: Evidence from latest regional and international student assessments. Paper presented at the 11th International Congress on Mathematical Education, Monterrey, Mexico.

Ma, X., & Kishor, N. (1997). Attitude towards self, social factors, and achievement in mathematics: A meta-analysis review. *Educational Psychology Review, 9,* 89–120.

Ma, X., & Klinger, D. (2000). Hierarchical linear modelling of student and school effects on academic achievement. *Canadian Journal of Education, 25,* 41–55.

Marks, G. (2006). Are between- and within-school differences in student performance largely due to socioeconomic background? Evidence from 30 countries. *Educational Research, 48,* 21–40.

Mathews, L. (2003). Babies overboard! The complexities of incorporating culturally relevant teaching into mathematics instruction. *Educational Studies in Mathematics,53,* 61–82.

Mcgraw, R., Lubienski, S., & Strutchens, M. (2006). A closer look at gender in NAEP mathematics achievement and affect data: Intersections with achievement, race/ethnicity, and socioeconomic status. *Journal for Research in Mathematics Education, 37,* 129–150.

Mills, R. (1998). *Grouping students for instruction in middle schools.* ERIC Digest. ERIC: ED419631.

Pianta, R. et al. (2008). Classroom effects on children's achievement trajectory in elementary school. *American Educational Research Journal, 45,* 365–397.

Povey, H., & Boylan, M. (1998). Working class students and the culture of mathematics classroom in the UK. In A. Olive & K. Newstead (Eds.), *Proceedings of the 22nd PME International Conference, 4,* 9–16.

Pozzi, S., Noss, R., & Hoyles, C. (1998). Tools in practice, mathematics in use. *Educational Studies in Mathematics, 36,* 105–122.

Roscigno, V., & Ainsworth-Parnell, J. (1999). Race, cultural capital, and educational resources: Persistent inequalities and achievement returns. *Sociology of Education, 72*, 158–178.

Seah, W. T. (2004). Shifting the lens of inquiry into the socialisation of mathematics teachers: Nature of value differences. In I. Putt, R. Faragher & M. McLean (Eds.), *Proceedings of the 27th Annual Conference of the Mathematics Education Research Group of Australasia, 2*, 501–508. Townsville: James Cook University.

Setati, M., & Adler, J. (2001). Between languages and discourses: Language practices in primary multilingual mathematics classrooms in South Africa. *Educational Studies in Mathematics Education, 43*, 243–269.

Setati, M. (2003). Language use in multilingual mathematics classes in South Africa. In N. A. Pateman, B. J. Dougherty, & J. T. Zilliox (Eds.), *Proceedings of the 27th PME International Conference, 4*, 151–158.

Stevenson, H., Lee, S., & Stigler, J. (1986). Mathematics achievement of Chinese, Japanese, and American Children. *Science, 231*, 693–699.

Stillman, G., & Balatti, J. (2001). Contribution of ethnomathematics to mainstream mathematics classroom practice. In B. Atweh, H. Forgasz, & B. Nebres (Eds.), *Sociocultural research on mathematics education: An international perspective* (pp. 313–328). Mahwah, NJ: Lawrence Erlbaum Associates.

Sullivan, P., Tobias, S., & Mcdonough. (2006). Perhaps the decision of some students to engage in learning mathematics in school is deliberate. *Educational Studies in Mathematics Education, 62*, 81–99.

TIMSS (2000). *Gender differences in achievement: IEA's Third International Mathematics and Science Study (TIMSS)*. Boston, MA: Boston College.

Vale, C., Leder, G., & Forgasz, H. (2003). Equity, mathematics learning and technology. In N. A. Pateman, B. J. Dougherty, & J. T. Zilliox (Eds.), *Proceedings of the 27th PME International Conference, 1*, 137–165.

Vithal, R., & Skovsmose, O. (1997). The end of innocence: A critique of 'ethnomathematics'. *Educational Studies in Mathematics Education, 34*, 131–158.

Watson, A., & de Geest, E. (2005). Principled teaching for deep progress: Improving mathematical learning beyond methods and materials. *Educational Studies in Mathematics, 58*, 209–234.

White, L. (1959). *The evolution of culture*. New York: McGraw-Hill.

Wilurg, K. (2003). Technology and the new meaning of educational equity.

Zevenbergen, R. (2001). Mathematics, Social class and linguistic capital: An analysis of mathematics classroom interactions. In B. Atweh, H. Forgasz, & B. Nebres, *Sociocultural research on mathematics education: An international perspective* (pp. 201–215). Mahwah, NJ: Lawrence Erlbaum Associates.

Chapter 5

Astiz, M. et al. (2002). Slouching towards decentralization: Consequences of globalization for curricular control in national education systems. *Comparative Education Review, 46*, 66–88.

Bankov, K. et al. (2006). Assessing between-school variation in educational resources and mathematics and science achievement in Bulgaria. *Prospects: Quarterly Review of Comparative Education, 36*, 447–473.

Darling-Hammond, L. et al. (2003). Building instructional quality: "inside-out" and "outside-in" perspectives on San Diego's school reform. Center for the Study of Teaching and Policy: A research report. ERIC document (ED499088).

Desmond, C. (2002). The politics of privatization and decentralization in global school reform: The value of equity claims for neoliberalism at the World Bank and in El Salvador, ERIC document no. ED468518.

Hook W., Bishop W., & Hook, J. (2007). A quality math curriculum in support of effective teaching for elementary schools. *Educational Studies in Mathematics, 65*, 125–148.

Jurdak, M. E. (1989). Religion and language as culture carriers and barriers in mathematics education. In C. Kietel (Ed.), *Mathematics, education and society (science and technology education, Document Series No. 35)* (pp. 12–14). Paris: UNESCO.

Marks, G. (2006). Are between- and within-school differences in student performance largely due to socioeconomic background? Evidence from 30 countries. *Educational Research, 48*, 21–40.

Ma, X., & Klinger, D. (2000). Hierarchical linear modelling of student and school effects on academic achievement. *Canadian Journal of Education, 25*, 41–55.

Opdenakkar, J. *et al.* (2002). The effects of schools and classes on mathematics achievement. *School Effectiveness & School Improvement, 13*, 399–427.

PISA. (2005). *School factors related to quality and equity: Results from PISA 2000.* OECD Publishing.

Chapter 6

Jurdak, M. E. (1989). Religion and language as culture carriers and barriers in mathematics education. In C. Kietel (Ed.), *Mathematics, education and society (science and technology education, Document Series No. 35)* (pp. 12–14). Paris: UNESCO.

Stevenson, H., Lee, S., & Stigler, J. (1986). Mathematics achievement of Chinese, Japanese, and American Children. *Science, 231*, 693–699.

Stigler, J., & Hiebert, J. (1999). The Teaching gap: Best ideas from the world's teachers for improving education in the class room. New York: Free Press.

Chapter 7

Chrostowski, S. (2004). Developing the TIMSS 2003 background questionnaires. In M. O. Martin, I. V. S. Mullis, & S. J. Chrostowski (Eds.), *TIMSS 2003 technical report.* Chestnut Hill, MA: Boston College.

Martin, O. (2005b). *TIMSS 2003 user guide for the international database-supplement 1.* Boston: Boston College.

Martin, O. (2005c). *TIMSS 2003 User guide for the international database-supplement 3.* Boston, MA: Boston College.

Chapter 12

Engeström, Y. (1999).Activity theory and individual and social transformation. In
    Y. Engeström, R. Miettinen, & R. -L. Punamaki (Eds.), *Perspctives on activity
    theory* (pp. 19–38). Cambridge: Cambridge University Press.
UNESCO. (2000). *The Dakar Framework for Action: Education for All – Meeting
    our Collective Commitments.* World Education Forum, Dakar, Senegal, 26–28
    April. http://www.unesco.org/education/efa/ed-for-all/dakfram_eng.shtml

Index

Breinigsville, PA USA
08 November 2009
227103BV00012BB/106/P